WELLES-TURNER MEMORIAL LIBRARY
GLASTONBURY, CT 06033

W9-BBE-853

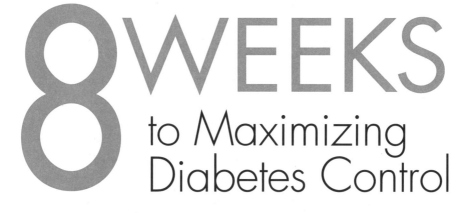

8WEEKS
to Maximizing Diabetes Control

HOW TO IMPROVE YOUR BLOOD GLUCOSE AND STAY HEALTHY WITH TYPE 2 DIABETES

Laura Hieronymus, MSEd, APRN, BC-ADM, CDE,
and
Christine Tobin, RN, MBA, CDE

DISCARDED BY
WELLES-TURNER MEMORIAL LIBRARY
GLASTONBURY, CT

In memory of
WILLIAM "SAM" KOWALSKY
and
DOROTHY S. KOWALSKY

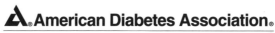

American Diabetes Association®
Cure • Care • Commitment®

Director, Book Publishing, Robert Anthony; *Managing Editor, Book Publishing,* Abe Ogden; *Editor,* Rebekah Renshaw; *Production Manager,* Melissa Sprott; *Composition,* pixiedesign llc; *Cover Design,* American Diabetes Association; *Printer,* United Graphics, Inc.

©2008 by the American Diabetes Association, Inc. All Rights Reserved. No part of this publication may be reproduced or transmitted in any form or by any means, electronic or mechanical, including duplication, recording, or any information storage and retrieval system, without the prior written permission of the American Diabetes Association.

Printed in the United States of America
1 3 5 7 9 10 8 6 4 2

The suggestions and information contained in this publication are generally consistent with the Clinical Practice Recommendations and other policies of the American Diabetes Association, but they do not represent the policy or position of the Association or any of its boards or committees. Reasonable steps have been taken to ensure the accuracy of the information presented. However, the American Diabetes Association cannot ensure the safety or efficacy of any product or service described in this publication. Individuals are advised to consult a physician or other appropriate health care professional before undertaking any diet or exercise program or taking any medication referred to in this publication. Professionals must use and apply their own professional judgment, experience, and training and should not rely solely on the information contained in this publication before prescribing any diet, exercise, or medication. The American Diabetes Association—its officers, directors, employees, volunteers, and members—assumes no responsibility or liability for personal or other injury, loss, or damage that may result from the suggestions or information in this publication.

♾ The paper in this publication meets the requirements of the ANSI Standard Z39.48-1992 (permanence of paper).

ADA titles may be purchased for business or promotional use or for special sales. To purchase this book in large quantities, or for custom editions of this book with your logo, contact Special Sales & Promotions, at the address below, or at booksales@diabetes.org or 703-299-2046.

American Diabetes Association
1701 North Beauregard Street
Alexandria, Virginia 22311

Library of Congress Cataloging-in-Publication Data

Hieronymus, Laura.
  8 weeks to maximizing diabetes control / Laura Hieronymus, Christine Tobin.
    p. cm.
  Includes index.
  ISBN 978-1-58040-279-8 (alk. paper)
  1. Diabetes--Popular works. I. Tobin, Christine. II. Title. III. Title: Eight weeks to maximizing diabetes control.

  RC660.4.H54 2008
  616.4'62--dc22

                        2008000957

Acknowledgments

*To my husband, G.D. (Chief), and our daughters,
Kelly and Lindsay, my life—my loves, for their support in
my ongoing efforts for diabetes education. —Laura*

*My gratitude to the people with diabetes who teach me
every day what it entails to fit diabetes into their lifestyles.
To my husband for his support. —Chris*

TABLE OF CONTENTS

"God grant me the serenity to accept the things I cannot change, the courage to change the things I can, and the wisdom to know the difference." —Reinhold Niebuhr

"Tell me and I'll forget. Show me and I'll remember. Involve me and I'll understand." —Confucius

"Nothing is particularly hard if you divide it into small jobs." —Henry Ford

"Ability is what you're capable of doing. Motivation determines what you do. Attitude determines how well you do it." —Lou Holtz

"We are what we repeatedly do. Excellence, therefore, is not an act but a habit." —Aristotle

FOREWORD

In the last 10 years, the number of new cases of type 2 diabetes has far exceeded experts' predictions. What used to be referred to as "adult-onset" diabetes—which primarily occurred in mid-to-later adulthood—is now being diagnosed in a much younger population, including children, adolescents, young adults, and women of child-bearing age. Among older adults over the age of 65, 20% have type 2 diabetes.

Persons with type 2 diabetes who cannot keep their blood glucose (sugar) levels in a healthy range are at a higher risk for serious and frequently life-threatening complications. The triple threat of poorly managed diabetes, uncontrolled blood pressure, and high cholesterol levels places those individuals at high risk for heart attacks and strokes. Also, blindness, kidney failure, and nerve disease often occur in persons who have not learned to properly manage their diabetes.

But it doesn't have to be that way. Diabetes complications can be prevented. Medical research has shown that by taking an active role in caring for your blood glucose levels, blood pressure, and cholesterol, you can potentially avoid these complications and live a full life.

You are the key member of your diabetes care team. Working closely with a team of health care professionals with expertise in medical care, dietary counseling, and teaching self-care skills is the best way to manage your diabetes and prevent complications from arising.

8 Weeks to Maximizing Diabetes Control combines current diabetes research with the authors' shared experience of over 40 years as certified diabetes educators. This book will provide a comprehensive and practical resource as you move forward in the quest to keep your blood glucose under the best possible control.

As health care professionals committed to excellence in diabetes care, we encourage you to stay educated, maintain a positive outlook, and always keep the advice of your diabetes care team close to your heart—LITERALLY!

John V. Borders, MD, FACP,
Internal Medicine Specialist

Edward I. Galaid, MD, MPH,
Internal Medicine/Preventive Medicine Specialist

Patti B. Geil, MS, RD, FADA, CDE,
Diabetes Nutrition Educator

Stacy D. Griffin, PharmD,
Diabetes Education Specialist

Kristina D. Humphries, MD,
Endocrinology and Metabolism Specialist

Carol B. Peddicord, MD,
Internal Medicine Specialist

INTRODUCTION

You can't change a diagnosis of diabetes. You are not the first person to wish that you didn't have diabetes, nor will you be the last. But the fact is, you do have diabetes and this chronic disease will be with you for the rest of your life. Life goes on…and the most important thing for you to do is learn how to get your blood glucose under control. The good news is that people with diabetes can learn to self-manage their disease. With type 2 diabetes, that generally means making some healthful changes in behavior to help control your blood glucose levels with the advice of your diabetes care team.

Whether you are newly diagnosed with type 2 diabetes or you have had it for several years, one thing is certain: Knowledge is power. The more you know about diabetes, the better equipped you are to make informed decisions about your health. You and your diabetes care team can work together to assure that you have the knowledge and skill that is necessary to help you attain and maintain the best possible blood glucose control. In addition, the ability to problem solve and have effective coping strategies to deal with the ups and downs of managing a chronic disease are necessary to achieve positive lifestyle behaviors. The American Association of Diabetes Educators developed a framework of seven self-care behaviors that measure, monitor, and manage outcomes.

AADE 7 SELF-CARE BEHAVIORS

The following self-care behaviors are the framework for measuring, monitoring, and managing outcomes.

1. Healthy eating
2. Being active
3. Monitoring
4. Taking medication
5. Problem solving
6. Healthy coping
7. Reducing risks

American Association of Diabetes Educators, AADE Self-Care Behaviors. www.diabeteseducator.org. Accessed March 2007.

8 Weeks to Maximizing Diabetes Control offers suggestions and guidance for people with diabetes to help put into perspective these diabetes self-management tasks or self-care behaviors that, at times, can seem overwhelming. It may be helpful for you to think about these self-care behaviors as they relate to your personal diabetes health.

Taking each self-care behavior and dividing it into realistic goals may help you move forward. To help maximize your diabetes control, you may want to focus on one self-care behavior and make changes in that area. Or in some cases, it may benefit you more to make changes that will enhance more than one self-care behavior to positively impact your blood glucose control. The eight-week format that is introduced with self-care behaviors that are strategic in diabetes management can be evaluated with your A1C measurements. Although the A1C is an index of average blood glucose for approximately 120 days, the preceding 30 days contribute more to the level of A1C than blood glucose levels 90–120 days prior.

As significant new research in the area of diabetes is published and more and more tools and technology are available, it always remains important for you to be aware of and embrace the variety of recommendations to enhance your diabetes health.

All the best,

Laura Hieronymus, MSEd, APRN, BC-ADM, CDE

Christine Tobin, RN, MBA, CDE

CHAPTER 1	Understanding Diabetes

Diabetes mellitus is a disorder of metabolism (or the breakdown of nutrients, primarily carbohydrates). Often just referred to as diabetes, it is characterized by higher than normal amounts of glucose (or sugar) in the bloodstream. The higher blood glucose levels are the result of the body's lack of insulin production or the inability to use the insulin that is present in the body. Insulin is a naturally occurring hormone that regulates the amount of glucose present in your bloodstream. Insulin is produced by the pancreas, which is about 6–10 inches in size and located in the body just behind the stomach. In a sense, diabetes is not a single disease, but rather a group of conditions that includes type 1, type 2, and gestational diabetes. There is also a condition called pre-diabetes, which almost always occurs before type 2 diabetes.

Type 1

Type 1 occurs when the body no longer produces or produces very little insulin. Although type 1 can occur at any age, it is most common in children and young adults. The vast majority of type 1 cases are caused by the autoimmune destruction of the pancreatic beta cells, which results in the inability to produce insulin. It is characterized by the rapid onset of symptoms, including weight loss and increased thirst, urination, and hunger. Because of the lack of insulin production by the body, those with type 1 diabetes require insulin therapy as part of their diabetes treatment plan.

Type 2

Type 2 is the most common form of diabetes, occurring in about 95% of those diagnosed with the disease. In type 2, the body typically produces insulin early on; however, your body has difficulty using the insulin properly. Type 2 diabetes is typically not diagnosed until

TYPE 2 DIABETES— HOW RISKY IS IT?

Type 2 diabetes accounts for the majority of cases of diabetes. In fact, it is estimated that of the 21 million Americans with diabetes, 19 million have type 2, with one-third of those being unaware that they have it. Individuals with the following characteristics are at risk for type 2 diabetes:

- A lack of physical activity in their daily life

- A first-degree relative with type 2 diabetes (mother, father, or sibling)

- A high-risk ethnicity (African American, Latino, Native American, Asian American, or Pacific Islander)

- A personal history of gestational diabetes

- Delivered a baby weighing more than 9 pounds

- High blood pressure

- A low HDL (good) cholesterol level or high triglyceride level

- Polycystic ovary syndrome (PCOS)

- A history of pre-diabetes

- Acanthosis nigricans (a condition characterized by darkening of the skin folds of the armpits, neck, or groin; usually associated with obesity)

- A history of vascular problems (disease of the blood vessels)

complications appear, which is the reason nearly one-third of cases are undiagnosed. Insulin resistance is usually present and it is believed that it often occurs first, followed by a decline in pancreatic function and insulin production. Type 2 can occur at any age, but is most common in those with one or more risk factors for the disease.

Gestational Diabetes

Gestational diabetes occurs exclusively during pregnancy and affects about 7% of all pregnancies in the United States. In most cases, blood glucose levels return to normal after pregnancy. Women who have had gestational diabetes are more likely to develop it with subsequent pregnancies, and are at higher risk for type 2 diabetes later in life.

Pre-diabetes

Pre-diabetes occurs when blood glucose levels are higher than normal, but not yet high enough to be diagnosed as diabetes. Pre-diabetes affects approximately

54 million people in the United States. People with prediabetes are 5–15 times more likely to develop type 2 diabetes than people with normal glucose values.

Diabetes Is Serious

According to a nationwide study conducted by the American Diabetes Association, only 32% of people perceived type 2 diabetes as a serious threat to their health. Keeping blood glucose levels in a near normal range has been shown to reduce the risk for complications of diabetes—such as eye, kidney, and nerve disease—but glucose levels are not the only concern in diabetes management. Along with the potential for high blood glucose levels, many individuals with type 2 have lipid (cholesterol and triglyceride) disorders, as well as hypertension (high blood pressure). If you have type 2 diabetes, this translates into a two to four times greater incidence of heart disease than those without diabetes. All of these concerns—blood glucose, blood pressure, and blood fats—should be addressed in a comprehensive treatment plan for optimal diabetes health outcomes.

PREVALENCE OF DIABETES IN THE U.S.
NOW UP TO 20.8 MILLION

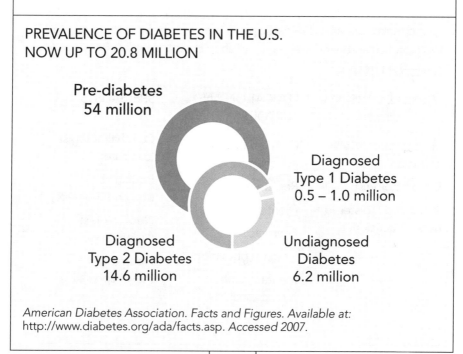

Pre-diabetes
54 million

Diagnosed
Type 1 Diabetes
0.5 – 1.0 million

Diagnosed
Type 2 Diabetes
14.6 million

Undiagnosed
Diabetes
6.2 million

American Diabetes Association. Facts and Figures. Available at: http://www.diabetes.org/ada/facts.asp. Accessed 2007.

Get Involved—Be a Part of Your Team

Dealing with diabetes day after day is a work in progress. You will have your work cut out for you, so don't do it alone. Research indicates that a team approach is the most effective route to treating and managing your diabetes. The primary goal of treatment is the best possible blood glucose control. You are the key team member and know your diabetes better than anyone. You are involved in carrying out the recommendations of your diabetes care team that will best treat your disease. Typical team members include your physician, a registered nurse, and registered dietitian (RD). Along with these health care professionals, your pharmacist and possibly a mental health professional round out the team for optimal diabetes care.

From time to time, you will need specialists on your team to help you with temporary issues. You may need a podiatrist if you have foot problems, or an obstetrician if you are a woman with diabetes

YOUR DIABETES DREAM TEAM

As an essential player on your diabetes care team, it is ultimately up to you to make sure all of the participants are present. Each team member has a particular role on the team and should work together for a common goal—your health.

MEDICAL CARE	EDUCATION AND SUPPORT	SPECIALISTS
Primary care physician	Certified diabetes educator (CDE)	Ophthalmologist (eye care)
Endocrinologist	Registered nurse	Podiatrist (toe and foot care)
Advanced registered nurse practicioner	Dietitian	Nephrologist (kidney specialist)
	Pharmacist	Neurologist (nerve specialist)
	Exercise physiologist	
	Mental health professional	

planning to become pregnant. Your diabetes care team may also refer you to an eye specialist, such as an ophthalmologist or optometrist, for a retinal exam.

Diabetes Self-Management Education

Diabetes self-management education is sometimes referred to as diabetes self-management training and is valuable because it helps you learn more about the disease. Diabetes educators are health care professionals who focus on helping people with diabetes understand their disease and learn how to adjust their lifestyle and behavior with self-management skills. A diabetes educator may be a nurse, dietitian, pharmacist, or other health care professional. These health care professionals can become certified in specific areas of expertise like diabetes education and management.

A certified diabetes educator (CDE) credential demonstrates that the health care professional possesses distinct and specialized knowledge about diabetes and its treatment. The board certified–advanced diabetes management (BC-ADM) certification is available only for registered nurses, dietitians, and pharmacists who also have an advanced degree. This certification recognizes that the health care professional has met certain predetermined standards specified by that profession for specialty practice. Its purpose is to ensure the public that an individual has mastered a body of knowledge and acquired skills and abilities in a particular specialty.

Some diabetes educators are also certified pump trainers, meaning they have completed a program designed by an insulin pump company to enhance their knowledge and expertise in the operation and training process for a specific brand of insulin pump.

In some cases, a health care provider may have more than one specialty certification that is diabetes focused, as well as other certifications that are not specific to diabetes.

CHAPTER 2 | Healthy Eating

Healthy eating is not a new concept. Health care professionals recommend healthy eating to all of their patients, so having diabetes is not a prerequisite for good nutrition. In reality, healthful eating plays a role in the prevention, as well as the treatment, of type 2 diabetes. In the Diabetes Prevention Program study, the most effective methods of preventing type 2 diabetes included a combination of making healthier food choices with a 7% weight loss (on average) and increasing physical activity to include 30-minute exercise sessions at least five days every week.

For people with diabetes, the American Diabetes Association has identified four primary goals for healthy nutrition:

- Achieving and maintaining blood glucose and blood pressure levels in the normal range, or as close to normal as safely possible, as well as a lipid (blood fat) profile that reduces the risk for blood vessel disease.

- Preventing (or slowing) development of diabetes-related complications by modifying nutrition intake and lifestyle behavior.

- Taking into account individual nutrition needs and willingness to change, as well as any personal and cultural preferences.

- Maintaining the pleasure of eating by limiting only those food choices indicated by scientific evidence.

Meal Planning

Meal planning can help you reach your blood glucose, blood pressure, and blood lipid goals while managing your diabetes. Adapting eating behaviors to balance carbohydrate intake throughout the day, along with making lower fat choices and controlling portion size, are the first steps in keeping your blood glucose, blood pressure, and blood lipid levels optimally controlled. Improvement in blood glucose control is proven to reduce the risk of long-term complications in type 2 diabetes.

Because food is such an important part of our lifestyle, as well as the cornerstone of diabetes management, you will want to take an aggressive approach to making the dietary changes that benefit your health. Gone are the days of buying special foods to meet your diabetes nutrition needs. You can eat the same foods that your entire family eats as long as you pay particular attention to the nutrition content and the portion size. Because type 2 diabetes has a genetic component, your relatives are also at risk, so your entire family will benefit from healthier eating.

An RD can work with you to determine a meal plan that is healthy, fits your preferences, and helps provide balance within your diabetes treatment plan. Studies show that working with a dietitian, and learning about medical nutrition therapy, can lower A1C levels by 1 to 2%. When you schedule the appointment, ask about insurance coverage for the service. Most insurance, including Medicare, will cover the visit if the dietitian is considered a provider of medical nutrition therapy or diabetes training.

There is no time like the present to start eating healthfully. You may feel that you have always tried to eat healthy but wonder why your blood glucose levels and your weight aren't what they used to be. Keep in mind that type 2 diabetes is a progressive disease and, although some natural insulin is typically present when you are diagnosed, insulin production and diabetes control may decline over time. At some point, medication may need to be added alongside your meal plan to maximize blood glucose control.

A-Weigh We Go

Two out of three people with type 2 diabetes are overweight and may want to work toward a healthier body weight. Weight patterns describe where excess weight is located on the body and are typically described as an apple versus a pear shape. An apple shape is

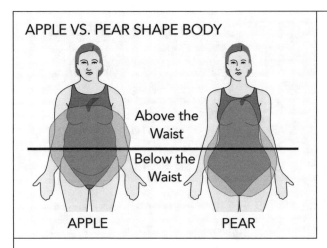

APPLE VS. PEAR SHAPE BODY

Above the Waist

Below the Waist

APPLE

PEAR

when more fat is distributed around the trunk or middle section of the body.

The apple shape is most common in type 2 diabetes, where excess weight is often concentrated in the central (middle) part of the body. This type of weight can interfere with metabolism and the breakdown of nutrients, and may cause issues with blood glucose and blood fat breakdown. Therefore, excess weight in this area of the body is more dangerous to your health than weight distributed in the pear shape.

Body mass index and waist circumference

The measurements that may be most useful to you as you get started are your body mass index (BMI) and waist circumference. Your BMI assesses your size in terms of your height and weight. BMI can help you understand how much total fat is in your body. A BMI of 25 or higher is considered overweight and a BMI of 30 or higher is considered a parameter for obesity.

To figure out your BMI, you will want to cross reference your height in inches to your weight in pounds in the table on page 10 and determine the BMI at the top of the table. For example, if you are 66 inches tall (5′6″) and weigh 192 pounds, then your BMI is 31. The BMI, according to the parameters above, indicate that this individual is obese.

Your waist circumference can help you figure out how much fat is around your middle section. To check your waist circumference, take a tape measure (one that is flexible and bends easily) and place it at your belly button, pulling it snugly around the body. The total

BODY MASS INDEX TABLE

	Normal						Overweight					Obese										Extreme Obesity														
BMI	19	20	21	22	23	24	25	26	27	28	29	30	31	32	33	34	35	36	37	38	39	40	41	42	43	44	45	46	47	48	49	50	51	52	53	54
Height (inches)												Body Weight (pounds)																								
58	91	96	100	105	110	115	119	124	129	134	138	143	148	153	158	162	167	172	177	181	186	191	196	201	205	210	215	220	224	229	234	239	244	248	253	258
59	94	99	104	109	114	119	124	128	133	138	143	148	153	158	163	168	173	178	183	188	193	198	203	208	212	217	222	227	232	237	242	247	252	257	262	267
60	97	102	107	112	118	123	128	133	138	143	148	153	158	163	168	174	179	184	189	194	199	204	209	215	220	225	230	235	240	245	250	255	261	266	271	276
61	100	106	111	116	122	127	132	137	143	148	153	158	164	169	174	180	185	190	195	201	206	211	217	222	227	232	238	243	248	254	259	264	269	275	280	285
62	104	109	115	120	126	131	136	142	147	153	158	164	169	175	180	186	191	196	202	207	213	218	224	229	235	240	246	251	256	262	267	273	278	284	289	295
63	107	113	118	124	130	135	141	146	152	158	163	169	175	180	186	191	197	203	208	214	220	225	231	237	242	248	254	259	265	270	278	282	287	293	299	304
64	110	116	122	128	134	140	145	150	157	163	169	174	180	186	192	197	204	209	215	221	227	232	238	244	250	256	262	267	273	279	285	291	296	302	308	314
65	114	120	126	132	138	144	150	156	162	168	174	180	186	192	198	204	210	216	222	228	234	240	246	252	258	264	270	276	282	288	294	300	306	312	318	324
66	118	124	130	136	142	148	155	161	167	173	179	186	192	198	204	210	216	223	229	235	241	247	253	260	266	272	278	284	291	297	303	309	315	322	328	334
67	121	127	134	140	146	153	159	166	172	178	185	191	198	204	211	217	223	230	236	242	249	255	261	268	274	280	287	293	299	306	312	319	325	331	338	344
68	125	131	138	144	151	158	164	171	177	184	190	197	203	210	216	223	230	236	243	249	256	262	269	276	282	289	295	302	308	315	322	328	335	341	348	354
69	128	135	142	149	155	162	169	176	182	189	196	203	209	216	223	230	236	243	250	257	263	270	277	284	291	297	304	311	318	324	331	338	345	351	358	365
70	132	139	146	153	160	167	174	181	188	195	202	209	216	222	229	236	243	250	257	264	271	278	285	292	299	306	313	320	327	334	341	348	355	362	369	376
71	136	143	150	157	165	172	179	186	193	200	208	215	222	229	236	243	250	257	265	272	279	286	293	301	308	315	322	329	338	343	351	358	365	372	379	386
72	140	147	154	162	169	177	184	191	199	206	213	221	228	235	242	250	258	265	272	279	287	294	302	309	316	324	331	338	346	353	361	368	375	383	390	397
73	144	151	159	166	174	182	189	197	204	212	219	227	235	242	250	257	265	272	280	288	295	302	310	318	325	333	340	348	355	363	371	378	386	393	401	408
74	148	155	163	171	179	186	194	202	210	218	225	233	241	249	256	264	272	280	287	295	303	311	319	326	334	342	350	358	365	373	381	389	396	404	412	420
75	152	160	168	176	184	192	200	208	216	224	232	240	248	256	264	272	279	287	295	303	311	319	327	335	343	351	359	367	375	383	391	399	407	415	423	431
76	156	164	172	180	189	197	205	213	221	230	238	246	254	263	271	279	287	295	304	312	320	328	336	344	353	361	369	377	385	394	402	410	418	426	435	443

Adapted from Clinical Guidelines on the Identification, Evaluation, and Treatment of Overweight and Obesity in Adults: The Evidence Report.

HEALTHY EATING

number of inches should be less than 35 inches for a woman and 40 inches for a man. If it is greater, there is too much weight in the middle section of your body. If your waist sags in the middle, your diabetes care prescriber may ask you to lie down prior to measuring your waist to help better determine the circumference.

What Should I Eat?

Asking the expert what you should eat is the best advice for dietary management in type 2 diabetes. No one person has the same eating habits, so the choices you make should be individualized to your likes and dislikes. When you make those choices, you should consider the main nutrients in the foods (carbohydrates, fat, and protein).

Nutrition experts recommend a healthful dietary pattern that includes carbohydrates from fruits, legumes, and low-fat milk. Carbohydrate-containing foods are important sources of energy, fiber, vitamins, and minerals. Limiting saturated and trans fat is vital to diabetes management because these types of fat contribute to low density lipoprotein (LDL) or "bad" cholesterol. Daily recommendations suggest limiting your consumption of cholesterol to less than 200 mg and making sure that less than 7% of your calories come from saturated fat. Dietary protein for those with diabetes is based on the same standards as the general population—about 15–20% of your daily calories.

Carbohydrate Awareness

Carbohydrates are the sugars and starches in the foods you eat. Regardless of the source, carbohydrates affect your blood glucose level more than protein or fat. Carbohydrates are broken down into blood glucose, which enters your bloodstream and causes your blood glucose level to rise after you eat. Although protein and fat don't affect blood glucose immediately, attention to fat intake is important for heart health when you have diabetes.

Because carbohydrate-containing foods affect blood glucose levels shortly after eating, be careful to avoid more carbohydrates than the body can handle at once. Many people with type 2 diabetes also take medication to help control blood glucose levels; therefore, it is important to understand how the medication works. Carbohydrate intake may be modified to work with a particular diabetes medication (see Chapter 5). Spreading carbohydrates out over the course of the day is a helpful strategy to keep fairly minimal amounts eaten at any given time and to help maintain blood glucose levels and prevent hunger.

My Pyramid

It will take some time but you will want to get a handle on the food sources that contain carbohydrates. Experts typically use the My Pyramid, the USDA's new food guide system, to help the general public (age 2 and older) determine patterns for eating. It is recommended, as discussed earlier, that those with a chronic condition—such as diabetes—consult with a health care provider to find the dietary plan that is the right one to meet their health needs. The My Pyramid is a specialized food guide system that determines how many servings of each food group you should consume each day depending on your age, sex, weight, height, and normal physical activity levels. Looking at the My Pyramid can give you a good idea of the various nutrients recommended in the meal plan.

Understanding what foods are considered sources of carbohydrates will help identify where carbs come from. The My Pyramid is divided into grains, vegetables, fruits, milk, meat and beans, and oils. To get your specialized food pyramid, ask your nutrition expert to assist you.

Grains

Any food made from wheat, rice, oats, cornmeal, barley, or other grains is a grain product. Bread, pasta, oatmeal, breakfast cereals, tortillas, and grits are examples of grain products. Fifteen grams of carbohydrate is typically considered a serving of these particular foods. Grains are divided into two subgroups: whole grains and refined grains. Whole grains contain the entire grain kernel, which includes the bran, germ, and endosperm. Some common examples include whole-wheat flour, cracked wheat, oatmeal, and brown rice.

Milling, or the process that removes the bran and germ, is the requirement for creating a refined grain. This is typically done to give the grains a finer texture and improve their shelf life, but it also removes dietary fiber, iron, and many B vitamins. Some examples of refined grains are white flour, white bread, and white rice. Many of the refined grains are enriched, which includes adding certain B vitamins (thiamin, riboflavin, niacin, folic acid) and iron back into the product after processing. Experts will usually recommend the whole grain over the refined grain since fiber is not added back into the refined product.

Vegetables

Any vegetable or 100% vegetable juice counts as a member of the vegetable group. Vegetables may be raw, cooked, fresh, frozen, canned, dried, or dehydrated and may be whole, cut up, or mashed. Vegetables are organized into 5 subgroups based on their nutrient content. The subgroups are dark green vegetables, orange vegetables, dry beans and peas, starchy vegetables, and other. It is important to know that the subgroups of dark green, orange, and other vegetables typically contain about 5 grams of carbohydrate for every 1 cup of raw and every 1/2 cup of cooked vegetables. These are considered "free" foods because they have very little impact on blood glucose control when eaten in reasonable serving amounts. The subgroups which contain dry beans and peas and starchy vegetables contain more total carbohydrates and must be accounted for in the meal plan. One-half cup of these two subgroups is typically about 15 grams of carbohydrates.

Fruits

Any fruit or 100% fruit juice counts as part of the fruit group. Fruits may be fresh, canned, frozen, or dried, and may be whole, cut up, or pureed. While fruits are fat free and contain healthy vitamins and minerals, they also contain carbohydrates. You will want to be attentive to your fruit intake and the total amount of carbohydrates in the foods that you eat. Common fruits eaten that are equivalent to 15 grams of carbohydrate include: a small apple (2 inches in diameter), a small banana (about 4 inches long), 1/2 cup (4 oz) orange juice, or 17 grapes.

Milk

All milk products and many foods made from milk are considered part of this food group. Foods made from milk that retain their calcium content are part of the group, while foods made from milk that have little or no calcium—such as cream cheese, cream, and butter—are not. The healthiest milk group choices are those that are fat free or low fat. Many of the foods from the milk group contain carbohydrates, such as milk and milk-based desserts like ice cream, ice milk, pudding, and yogurt products. An 8-oz glass of milk is about 12 grams of carbohydrates. Checking the nutrition facts label is key to helping you determine total carbohydrate content, as well as maintaining your awareness of the fat content for these items. Cheese is another product that contains milk, however, it is generally lower in carbohydrates per serving.

Meat and beans

All foods made from meat, poultry, fish, eggs, nuts, legumes, and seeds are considered part of the meat and beans group. These foods contain very little, if any, carbohydrates. Dry beans and peas are part of the meat and beans group as well as the vegetable group because they may be regularly substituted for meat (as a protein substance) by those individuals who eat very little or no meat. Dry beans and peas do contain carbohydrates and need to be counted. Most meat and poultry choices should be lean or low fat. Fish, nuts, and seeds contain healthy oils, so choose these foods frequently instead of meat or poultry.

A key to eating healthy is to make changes you can live with. In other words, diabetes is around for life and since healthy eating is a part of your treatment plan, your goal should be to learn strategies that work best for you. Divide and conquer! Think about and move forward with the changes you want to make—keeping in mind the week by week suggestions mentioned here.

Perhaps the best place to start is figuring out what you are eating now. Successful weight-loss programs ask individuals to be accountable for what they eat. One way to accomplish this is to keep a diary of foods eaten on a daily basis and then review the records to determine what, how much, and when you are eating. Sharing your food diary with your RD may be a helpful way to create problem-solving strategies to make healthier choices. To get started, include the following information as you track your food intake:

- Date
- Time you eat
- Food consumed (including all food, all day long)
- Amount of food eaten (as close as possible)
- Reason for eating
- Total carbohydrate content
- Calorie intake

Date

Along with the date, write down the day of the week. Do you see any trends on certain days of the week? For example, does your food intake change the busier you are? If so, how does it change? As you write down the amounts of food you are eating, are you surprised? As the days go by, do you see yourself changing your intake at all?

Time you eat

Are you taking time for breakfast? How often are you eating on a daily basis? Did you realize when and how often you were eating (or not eating)?

Food consumed

Be specific about the types of food you eat. For example, if you have a slice of bread, what kind of bread—White? Whole wheat? Whole grain? Honey wheat? This can help you and your dietitian better evaluate how nutritious your choices are.

Amount of food eaten

Be as honest and specific as possible. Use a measuring cup and spoons to determine the number of servings in a packaged food to be as accurate as possible.

Reason for eating

Add comments about the reason you are eating any amount of food. Are you hungry? Is everyone else eating (one, two, or three servings) and does that influence you? Do you eat when you feel nervous? Bored? Depressed? Do you eat when you watch television?

Total carbohydrate content

It may be helpful for you to track the carbohydrate content in terms of the number of carbohydrate choices in a particular food (one choice = 15 grams of total carbohydrates), or simply the total number of grams of carbohydrate in the item consumed. Tracking carbohydrates may help you create an awareness of total carbohydrate content in foods that you typically eat, and determine if you are consistent with carbo-hydrates from meal to meal.

Calorie intake

In many cases, monitoring calories can be beneficial. You may find that some of your favorite foods are loaded with calories. While you might not be willing to totally give up these foods, perhaps you might be willing to eat them less frequently, or in smaller amounts, if it means making positive changes toward better health. You may find that some foods are higher in calories than you suspected, or that by taking some steps to modify a recipe you can lower the fat and calorie amounts without sacrificing the good taste. By looking at your caloric comparison from day to day, you may notice patterns to help you make decision that can improve overall calorie consumption and provide better consistency in caloric amounts on a daily basis. Also, the information can create an awareness of the nutrition content, as well as the portion sizes, of the foods you are eating.

It is a known fact that carbohydrates are the nutrients that most directly influence blood glucose levels. As a person with diabetes, you need to know the target amount of total carbohydrates as you work with your meal planning. Work together with your RD to determine the healthiest number of carbohydrate grams with each meal and snack that you eat. By considering your age, body weight, activity level, any other medical problems you might have, as well as any desire you have to lose weight, the two of you can set up a plan that you can live with.

KEEPING CARBS CONSISTENT

Using the table below, find the adult that best describes you. Try and stay as close as possible to the number of grams of total carbohydrate listed for each meal and snack. Spreading carbohydrates out through the day can help minimize the load in your body at any given time. Snacks can help prevent hunger from meal to meal. This information does not replace expert advice. The best plan is one developed by you and your RD.

	Breakfast	Mid-morning	Lunch	After-noon	Dinner	Bedtime	Total Carbs
Anyone wanting to lose weight	45	15	45	15	45	15	180
Older Women	45	15	45	15	45	15	180
Women	45	15	45	15	60	15	195
Larger women, older men	60	15	45	15	60	15	210
Active women, most men	60	15	60	15	75	15	240
Active men	90	15	75	15	90	15	300

(Carbs counted in grams.)
Adapted from A Field Guide to Type 2 Diabetes. *American Diabetes Association, 2004.*

To get started until you see the RD, set a target to maintain as consistent of a carbohydrate intake as possible. As you begin to have questions about your meal planning, keep notes so your RD can help you better understand your meal planning effort. Keep in mind that meal planning is an important part of your treatment plan, so don't look upon it lightly. Just as you would follow up with your physician if he prescribed a medication for you, be sure you do the same with the RD. Follow-up visits with the RD can help you get your carbohydrate and nutrition needs adjusted to help you get the best possible glucose control.

Nutrition labeling of foods is required by the Food and Drug Administration (FDA), under the Nutrition Labeling and Education Act of 1990—which identifies the nutrients that must be listed on food labels, other ingredients that may be listed, health claims, and standard portion sizes. The Act also defines terminology commonly used on labels such as light, low fat, and sodium free. The nutrition information on food labels can be found in several locations—the nutrition facts panel, the ingredients list, and other areas of the label where health claims may be displayed. As a consumer with diabetes, skill at reading food labels and recognizing the nutrient content of foods may benefit your blood glucose control.

Your best source of information is the nutrition facts panel, where manufacturers provide serving size information, quantities of specific nutrients, and percent Daily Values (%DV). Nutrient information required on all food labels includes total calories, calories from fat, total fat, saturated fat, trans fat, cholesterol, sodium, total carbohydrate, dietary fiber, sugars, protein, vitamin A, vitamin C, calcium, and iron.

BASIC NUTRITION LABEL

Nutrition Facts

Serving Size 1 cup (228g)
Servings Per Container 2

Amount Per Serving

Calories 260   **Calories from Fat** 120

	% Daily Value*
Total Fat 13g	**20%**
Saturated Fat 5g	**25%**
Trans Fat 2g	
Cholesterol 30mg	**10%**
Sodium 660mg	**28%**
Total Carbohydrate 31g	**10%**
Dietary Fiber 0g	**0%**
Sugars 5g	
Protein 5g	

Vitamin A 4%	•	Vitamin C 2%
Calcium 15%	•	Iron 4%

*Percent Daily Values are based on a 2,000 calorie diet. Your Daily Values may be higher or lower depending on your calorie needs.

	Calories:	2,000	2,500
Total Fat	Less than	65g	80g
Sat Fat	Less than	20g	25g
Cholesterol	Less than	300mg	300mg
Sodium	Less than	2,400mg	2,400mg
Total Carbohydrate		300g	375g
Dietary Fiber		25g	30g

Calories per gram:
Fat 9 • Carbohydrate 4 • Protein 4

Check the serving size

All of the information on the nutrition facts panel reflects the serving size listed in the print.

Calories

The calorie information tells you the number of calories in the serving size (serving size listed on the nutrition facts panel). If the serving size is increased, then the calorie amount is increased; likewise, if the serving size is cut in half, then the calorie amount is 50% less.

Limit the fat

The American Diabetes Association recommends that people limit their saturated fat intake to less than 7% of total calories, along with a minimal intake of trans fat, on a daily basis. Saturated fat is a fat or oil—from either animal or vegetable sources—that is typically solid at room temperature. Eating foods high in saturated fat is thought to contribute to higher levels of cholesterol in the blood. Trans fats are partially saturated and may increase your risk of heart disease. Your dietary cholesterol intake should be <200 mg on a daily basis and your overall daily fat intake should be determined based on your individual need. Expert counseling with an RD is important to learn more about the various types of fat, as well as a recommended total daily intake of fat that is right for you.

Check the total carbohydrate

Focus on total carbohydrate (sugar is only part of the total carbohydrates) to determine the amount of carbohydrates in a serving. The total carbohydrates listed on the nutrition facts label are 31 grams for each 1 cup serving that you eat. If the serving size is changed, you should calculate the total carbohydrate to match the change. For example, if you eat 1/2 cup, then the total carbohydrate is 15 1/2 grams; likewise, for 2 cups, the total carbohydrate is 62 grams.

Note your protein

The amount of protein you need is based on your size, calorie needs, and stage of life. The ADA recommends that most adults get between 15 to 20% of their daily calorie requirement from protein. In general, men need about 60 grams of protein per day and women need about 45–50 grams of protein.

What about sodium?

Keep in mind that the ADA recommends that adults get about 2,400 mg of sodium on a daily basis. Use this as a guide when keeping track of daily sodium intake. In some cases, a restriction of sodium is recommended by your physician or RD. Adjust accordingly as you track the amount of sodium you eat.

While this information can help you get started, keep in mind that visits with an RD can help you further analyze the nutrition information on the foods you are eating and help you make healthy food choices to keep your blood glucose control optimal.

Whether it was in your early childhood years, any previous experience monitoring your eating habits, or any consults you have had in the past with a nutrition expert, somewhere down the line you have probably been exposed to portion sizes. These days, portion sizes are often blurred in a food service industry where smalls have become talls, mediums have become grandes, and larges are now super supremes. True, you may justify this by thinking you get more for your money, but in reality, increased portion sizes mean higher calories and more carbohydrates and fat, which can subsequently affect your blood glucose control and weight. Since weight is a concern of many with type 2 diabetes, sizing up your servings makes sense.

While portion sizes in the marketplace have increased, standard serving sizes found on food labels and used by RDs when designing diabetes meal plans have not. When working toward keeping your portions in check, the following tips may be helpful.

Measure your foods

If you want to be sure of how much you are eating, use measuring tools—such as measuring cups, spoons, or a food scale that measures food in grams. Start by putting your usual serving on a plate, in a bowl, or in a cup, and then measure it. Next, measure out the standard serving or the portion specific to your meal plan and compare. What is the difference? Are these changes you are willing to make? Keep in mind that YOU have to make the effort to scale down portion sizes.

Estimate food portions

While measuring food is by far the most accurate, there will be times when carting around measuring cups and spoons is not practical. In those instances, it may be helpful to use a measuring tool always available to you in any situation—your hands. Another way to help you estimate your portions is by using common, standard size items, such as tennis balls or a deck of cards. Learn to visualize these items when keeping your portions in check when measuring tools aren't an option. Examples include:

- 2 Tbsp peanut butter (ping-pong ball)

- 3 oz meat or poultry (deck of cards)

- 1 medium fruit (a tennis ball)

- 1/2 cup of fresh fruit (1/2 baseball)

- 1 1/2 oz of low-fat or fat-free cheese (4 stacked dice)

WONDERING HOW MUCH TO EAT? DO THE "HAND JIVE"!

Hand Jive is based on a method used in Zimbabwe where teaching without any written materials is a common approach. The hand teaching method is very useful for anyone when estimating portion sizes.

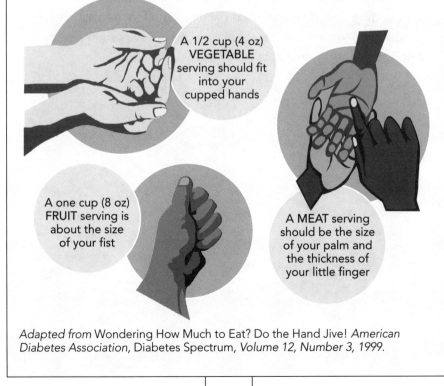

A 1/2 cup (4 oz) **VEGETABLE** serving should fit into your cupped hands

A one cup (8 oz) **FRUIT** serving is about the size of your fist

A **MEAT** serving should be the size of your palm and the thickness of your little finger

Adapted from Wondering How Much to Eat? Do the Hand Jive! *American Diabetes Association*, Diabetes Spectrum, *Volume 12, Number 3, 1999.*

Pre-portioned foods

Taking time in advance to package your foods in single portion sizes may be helpful. For example, measuring snack type foods and putting them in snack-size bags in 15 gram (carbohydrate) serving portions may be helpful in preventing the tendency to overeat, as well as keeping serving sizes in check. On pre-packaged foods, take time to review the nutrition facts label or ask your RD to help you figure out how to fit pre-portioned foods, such as frozen meals, into your meal plan.

Share a meal

Scale down the super size by requesting smaller portions when eating out. Appetizer portions may be smaller, so don't be shy about ordering from the appetizer menu. Adding a green salad or side of vegetables can be healthful. Share a meal with yourself by requesting the doggy bag at the start of the meal and saving some food for later. Take appropriate portion sizes from the plate and then store the rest to take home (even if you don't want to take it home, it helps to remove the excess food and avoid the temptation to overeat). Taking the steps to reverse the trend of ever-increasing portion sizes can help you tune up your eating habits and your health.

As you embark on your carbohydrate journey, think about the healthiest choices possible. For example, if you drink a serving (8 oz) of milk three times a day, you can save 180 calories a day by simply choosing skim milk over whole milk. That translates into 1,260 calories a week. An 8-oz serving of fat-free milk is approximately 90 calories, while an 8-oz serving of whole milk is about 150 calories. Do the math. Making low-fat choices in the appropriate serving sizes can mean fewer calories and help you meet your weight goals. What other choices can you make to keep calories in check?

TAKING THE FIRST STEP: HOW MANY CARBOHYDRATES DO I NEED?

Nutrition experts recommend that about half the calories you eat come from carbohydrates. One gram of carbohydrate contains about 4 calories, so if your daily meal plan contains 1,200 calories, that's about 600 calories or 150 grams of carbohydrate per day. (See week 2 to help balance total carbohydrate amounts through the day with meals and snacks.)

Calculate your daily calorie needs:

Your weight in pounds: _____

multiplied by your activity factor (as determined by the chart below): x _____

equals the number of calories you need each day to maintain your weight: = _____

Activity Factor

Very inactive, always dieting, waist circumference > 40 in.	10
Older than age 55, active woman, inactive man	13
Very active woman, active man	15
Very active man or athlete	20

To lose 1 pound a week, subtract 500 calories from the total number of calories needed each day. To lose 2 pounds a week, subtract 1,000 calories from the total number of calories needed each day.

Sample Meal Plan: _____ calories
(about 50% should come from carbohydrate)

Breakfast: _____ Carbohydrates

Midmorning Snack: _____ Carbohydrates

Lunch: _____ Carbohydrates

Mid-afternoon Snack: _____ Carbohydrates

Supper: _____ Carbohydrates

Bedtime Snack: _____ Carbohydrates

(Carbohydrates measured in grams.)

© DiabetesCare & Communications. Used with permission (2008).

You may be concerned about the amount of sugar you are eating and rightfully so. When you check a food label, the amount of sugar can give you important clues on how healthy a food is. Foods that contain a great deal of sugar are not typically the best nutritional choice because they don't usually contain a lot of fiber, vitamins, and minerals. In some cases, foods high in sugar are also high in fat content. While knowing the content of sugar is an important fact to note, you will still want to focus on the total carbohydrate content of foods with regard to blood glucose control.

Fat free doesn't necessarily mean calorie free. In many cases, fat-free foods are just as high in calories as the regular kind. When manufacturers remove the fat from an item, it is usually replaced with sugar, which translates to carbohydrates and adds to your total carbohydrate intake. Take fat-free salad dressings, for example. A common brand of fat-free ranch dressing is 30 calories, 0 fat grams, and 6 grams of total carbohydrate for a 2 Tbsp serving. The regular (same brand) ranch dressing has 140 calories per serving, 14 grams of fat (no trans or saturated fat), and 2 grams of total carbohydrate. The one with the lowest calorie content is the fat free; however, you may prefer the regular ranch dressing in regard to taste. The carbo-hydrate content is three times greater in the fat-free version because the soybean oil (a thickening agent that is primarily fat) is replaced with corn syrup (primarily sugar). Neither is a wrong choice, but it is important to know how it will affect your overall meal plan.

It is no small task to try and eat healthy meal after meal, day after day. Add a challenge like eating out, whether it's at a restaurant or at someone's home, and it gets very tough. In fact, the average American eats four or more meals away from home each week. You will need to be creative at times to make sure you are making the healthiest choices a majority of the time. Start with these tips to help you stay on the healthy side of eating when dining away from home.

Keep an open mind when menu gazing

Take a look at what the menu has to offer and compare the food items. Which might be a healthier choice? Don't be shy about asking the host or food server about a particular food, such as how it is prepared, and what sauces and spices are included. You are the customer so speak up; you have the right to know!

What is your pattern for eating out?

Start by taking a look at how often you eat out and why. Review the places that you tend to eat out and decide what control you have over the preparation of food.

Is nutrition information available?

Many restaurants have nutrition information for the food choices they provide. More often than not, the information is not posted at the place of dining, but may be available when requested or posted on the restaurant's website. The American Diabetes Association has books and other publications that address issues concerning dining out. Do your homework to figure out what foods are healthiest for you before you get to the restaurant!

Focus on your meal plan

Think about the recommendations that your RD has made and stay focused on trying to meet those goals. Learn to order items that can jeopardize your healthy eating—creamy sauces, heavy salad dressings, and condiments like sour cream and butter—on the side. Be careful and limit these types of foods or, if you are willing, just leave them out!

Stay within your limits

Review the portion size information and stay within your limits. This will go a long way to keeping your calories to the minimum. Many of us grew up thinking we couldn't leave the table until every morsel of food was eaten. It is best to always stay aware of the portion sizes when you order and keep overdoing it to a minimum.

Plan for events with never-ending food

Parties, restaurants, get-togethers, and picnics often have unlimited food available for extended periods of time. Don't let the buffet wear down your healthy outlook and your blood glucose control.

BUFFET TABLE TIPS

- Look for the high-fiber, low-fat options such as beans, peas, lentils, and dark green vegetables like broccoli, cabbage, spinach, and kale. Go for the bean salads and pasta salads that are primarily fresh vegetables. Make whole-grain choices like brown rice, couscous, whole-wheat bread, and pasta.

- Watch out for dishes loaded with fat—those with mayonnaise, sour cream, and butter. Choose veggies that are light on salad dressings and heavy sauces. Bring your own healthy version of salad dressing.

- Choose grilled or roasted meats over fried versions. Try and make lean choices (removing the skin if present).

- Choose fresh fruit and lighter options over cakes and pastries. Desserts are usually plentiful, so make the healthiest choice.

- Drink plenty of water. Iced tea with no added sugar and sugar-free soda are reasonable choices. If you choose to drink alcohol, stay in control. Generally, moderation is considered one alcoholic beverage for a woman and two for a man.

- Stay in carbohydrate control. Many healthy foods contain carbohydrates, so be sure and keep your targets in mind.

Adapted from Buffet Table Tips for People with Diabetes. Control Your Diabetes for Life (November 2005). http://www.ndep.nih.gov or http://www.cdc.gov/diabetes . Accessed February 2007.

You are human and are not perfect. With that in mind, take the time to recognize every positive change that you have made—maybe even make a list of those positive changes to recognize your accomplishments. Are you recognizing portion sizes by paying attention to them? Are you making healthier carbohydrate choices? How are you doing with eating out? Each small change that you make adds up, and everything you do to establish healthful eating is important.

How will you know if your healthy eating changes have made a difference in your diabetes control? Ask yourself the following: Do you feel better? How do you feel about yourself? Are you at a comfortable weight for you? What is your A1C?

Your diabetes team can request an A1C test, which gives a snapshot of blood glucose control over the previous 2 to 3 months. The lower your A1C, the better your chances are of avoiding serious diabetes complications. According to the American Diabetes Association, the recommended A1C goal for adults with diabetes is less than 7%, while an A1C level as close to normal (less than 6%) as possible is encouraged.

Healthful eating, along with physical activity and diabetes medicines, if needed, can help keep your blood glucose in target range. Take what you have learned and put it to good use. Your diabetes health outcome can only benefit from healthful eating.

CHAPTER 3	Being Active—The Magic of Movement

Being more active on a daily basis improves your overall physical health. Individuals who exercise regularly report increased self-esteem, reduced stress, and enhanced clarity of thought—who would argue with that? Routine physical activity also improves your confidence in your ability to make a behavior change. No matter what type of exercise and physical activity you choose to do, all of it counts toward better health outcomes.

What's in It for Diabetes?

Not only does being more physically active actually prevent diabetes, it offers the benefit of improving diabetes control by lowering blood glucose readings and decreasing body fat. The benefits of physical activity include weight control, and when moderate-to-intense aerobic physical activity is done regularly, the risk for cardiovascular disease declines. In fact, the American Diabetes Association recommends exercise and physical activity as an essential part of the treatment plan for type 2 diabetes.

People with type 2 diabetes have insulin resistance, where

HEALTH BENEFITS OF EXERCISE: THE BOTTOM LINE

- Preserves mobility, strength, and balance
- Increases bone density and strength
- Boosts brainpower and memory
- Reduces the risk of certain cancers
- Reduces cravings for alcohol, nicotine, caffeine, and sugar
- Improves insulin sensitivity, decreasing cardiometabolic risks
- May improve fibrinolysis (dissolving of blood clots)
- May prevent progression of type 2 diabetes
- Improves overall psychological well-being

muscle, fat, and liver cells do not respond normally to insulin. As a result, it takes more insulin than normal to get glucose into the cells for energy. Exercise can benefit the body by improving sensitivity to insulin, helping the body use insulin better. Since lipids (blood fat levels) and blood pressure are a concern to those people with type 2 diabetes, improvement in exercise can translate into lower total cholesterol, LDL (bad) cholesterol, and triglyceride levels, as well as lower blood pressure. Exercise has also been found to improve HDL (good) cholesterol levels, which is added protection against heart disease.

The Magic of Movement

The 1996 report of the Surgeon General states that for the general adult population: "…significant health benefits can be obtained by including a moderate amount of physical activity (30 minutes of brisk walking or raking leaves, 15 minutes of running, or 45 minutes of playing volleyball), on most days of the week." The report outlines a moderate amount of physical activity equivalent to any activity that burns 150 calories of energy per day, or 1,000 calories per week, with greater health benefits achieved by increasing the amount (duration, frequency, or intensity) of physical activity.

For those individuals with diabetes who are not able to set aside at least 30 minutes at a time for physical activity, research has shown that your heart and lung fitness gains are similar when your physical activity occurs in several short sessions—10 minute increments three times daily—as when the same total amount and intensity of activity occurs in one 30 minute session. The goal is to accumulate physical activity over the course of the day. So, washing windows can be as important as water aerobics to improving your overall fitness efforts.

The American Diabetes Association Standards of Medical Care include the types of exercise based on the 1996 report of the Surgeon General, in which the following definitions are outlined in physical activity and health.

Physical activity

Physical activity is defined as bodily movement produced by the contraction of skeletal muscle that requires energy expenditure in excess of resting energy expenditure. This includes any activity that keeps you moving—walking across the parking lot and going up (and down) a staircase are two examples of physical activity.

Exercise

Exercise is a subset of physical activity: planned, structured, and repetitive bodily movements performed to improve or maintain one or more component of physical fitness. Types of exercise include aerobic and resistance training. Anytime you go from being sedentary to pursuing an exercise program, it is essential that you talk with your diabetes care team on how to get started.

Aerobic exercise

Aerobic exercise consists of rhythmic, repeated, and continuous movements of the same large muscle groups for at least 10 minutes at a time, and includes walking, bicycling, jogging, swimming, and water aerobics, and playing most sports.

An effective physical activity program includes a proper warm up and cool down period along with the aerobic period. It is especially important for people with diabetes to take time to warm up, stretch, and cool down to improve their flexibility and to lower their risk for heart problems.

- The warm up prepares the muscles, heart, and lungs for more vigorous activity. A good warm up starts with 5–10 minutes of low-level aerobic activity, such as walking or cycling.

- Gentle stretching for 5–10 minutes follows the warm up. The stretches should include the muscles that will be used during the upcoming active portion of the workout.

- After warming up and stretching the muscles, your body is ready for the aerobic exercise portion. Aerobic exercise is exercise that raises your heart rate and requires an increase in oxygen over an extended period of time, which exercises the heart and lungs, as well as burning fat. Examples of aerobic exercise include brisk walking, running or jogging, swimming, cross-country skiing, ice skating, cycling, rollerblading, jumping rope, water aerobics, and aerobic dance.

- Following the aerobic portion is the cool down period. The 5–10 minute cool down should bring the heart rate down to pre-exercise level. Appropriate cool down activities include light or easy aerobic activity. Static stretching of the warmed up muscles can also be included at this point of the workout.

RESISTANCE TRAINING: SAFETY FIRST

Safety is always the best policy for your diabetes health. These are some basic guidelines and safety precautions for a person with diabetes who wants to start a weight-training program:

✓ Check with your diabetes care team before starting a resistance (weight) training program. You and your team will want to address any issues with your diabetes and blood glucose control.

✓ Start with lighter weights and higher repetition while concentrating on your form. A personal trainer may help you tailor the program to your needs and make sure you are using proper form.

✓ DO NOT hold your breath when you lift weights. This technique (known as the Valsalva maneuver) raises blood pressure and increases the pressure within your eyes.

✓ Always have a spotter if you are using free weights.

✓ Avoid any exercise that causes pain. Some soreness and burning in the actual muscle may occur; however, any exercise that causes a sharp or shooting pain or joint pain should be avoided.

Philbin, R. Weight Training and Diabetes: Safety Precautions Table. September 2005.

Resistance exercise

Resistance training consists of activities that use muscular strength to move a weight or work against a resistive load and includes weight lifting and exercises using weight machines. Resistance training can help you maintain a leaner body mass, helping with weight management.

For people with diabetes, resistance or weight training helps lower blood glucose levels by increasing the amount of glucose uptake in the muscles and helping the body store glucose. Your metabolism can benefit from resistance training by helping you burn more calories. Before you get started, consult with your diabetes care team to see if resistance training is right for you. It is best to consult with an expert in this field to assure the best possible outcomes along with safety.

It is important to understand the types and benefits of exercise and their relationship to your overall diabetes health. Developing a safe activity program should take into consideration your age, general health, level of diabetes control, diabetes medications, condition of your heart and circulatory system, and any diabetes-related complications you have. It is always recommended that you and your diabetes care team collaborate on the plan.

Understanding the FITT in Fitness

The American College of Sports Medicine has developed the FITT principle as a way to structure fitness goals to improve health and well-being. When you plan an exercise program, it is best to keep these factors in mind.

F is for **frequency** or how many times you will exercise on a weekly basis.

I is for **intensity** or how vigorously you should do an exercise.

T is for **time** or how long you should spend exercising.

T is for the **types** of exercise that you will do.

The appropriate frequency, intensity, time, and type of physical activity vary by individuals depending on their age, overall general health, as well as any diabetes-related complications. Your individual health and fitness goals, as well as your particular preference regarding exercise options, should always be considered. By doing something you like, your exercise efforts will continue for the long term.

It is important to think about making changes you can live with as you think about your physical activity and exercise efforts. Since your diabetes is here to stay, you may want to consider adding a physical activity and exercise regimen that you actually enjoy. You will probably be more likely to stick with it. As adults, we seem to always be short on time, so finding a friend or partner to support you with your ongoing efforts can be an easy way to help stick with it.

Start by determining your ability, based on your diabetes history, then develop the strategies for motivation and strive to keep a positive attitude. Move forward with the changes you want to make and you'll be on the road to positive lifestyle changes.

When you have a chronic illness like diabetes, it is important that you meet with your physician prior to making significant changes in your activity levels. In some cases, there may be limitations or restrictions to your exercise plan, or your physician may recommend formal exercise testing if you have been sedentary. It is also best to see your doctor first if you are at moderate to high risk for cardiovascular disease and are interested in adding an exercise program that is considered vigorous and would exceed the demands of your typical everyday living.

Undergoing formal exercise testing can help identify the presence of underlying heart and blood vessel problems before you embark on the exercise trail. If you are relatively healthy and are planning a moderate-intensity activity like walking, your physician may feel it is safe for you to get started without testing. If you have diabetes-related complications—such as eye disease, kidney disease, or nerve damage—your physician may make some suggestions about the type of exercise that is best for you.

Blood glucose control can be enhanced with regular physical activity and exercise; however, be cautious to avoid hypoglycemia (blood glucose levels that are too low). If you suffer from hyperglycemia (blood glucose levels that are too high) at the start of exercise, you may have to delay your plans until your blood glucose levels are closer to recommended ranges.

Hypoglycemia

Hypoglycemia is not as common during physical activity in people with type 2 diabetes as those with type 1, particularly if they don't take blood glucose-lowering medicines that have the side effect of hypoglycemia. The effect of exercise on your blood glucose level depends on many factors, including the time of day you plan to exercise, the timing of your diabetes medicines, when you ate, and how often and intensely you exercise. If you plan to exercise vigorously or for 45 minutes or more, then you may need to eat an additional 15–30 grams of carbohydrates to prevent hypoglycemia and keep blood glucose levels balanced. Usually your diabetes care team will recommend that you delay exercise if your blood glucose levels are too low prior to exercise plans.

Symptoms of hypoglycemia are caused by the brain's lack of glucose, or by the hormones, primarily epinephrine, that are released by the body to help increase blood glucose levels. For people with diabetes, a blood glucose level of 70mg/dL or less is usually considered low, with treatment being recommended to prevent blood glucose from becoming even lower. Warning signs of hypoglycemia are:

- Weakness

- Shakiness

- Sweatiness or clamminess

- Rapid heart rate

- Hunger

As blood glucose gets lower, the brain suffers from this lack of glucose, leading to trouble concentrating, changes in vision, slurred speech, loss of coordination, headaches, dizziness, and drowsiness. Mood changes may occur and can result in feelings of nervousness, being argumentative or aggressive, and even crying.

Treating hypoglycemia should be prompt. In some cases, people with diabetes are unable to recognize hypoglycemia in the early stages, which is called hypoglycemia unawareness. This can cause problems with making sure that treatment occurs in a timely manner, especially if a person progresses to confusion, which can then impair his or her ability to treat the hypoglycemia. People with hypoglycemia unawareness, those who are elderly or live alone, as well as young children are often given higher target goals for treating hypoglycemia

TREATMENT FOR HYPOGLYCEMIA

To treat hypoglycemia, you will want to check your blood glucose to confirm the level. If your blood glucose is at or below your target level, treat with 15 grams of carbohydrates. Some good carbohydrates to have on hand are:

- 3–4 glucose tablets
- 1 dose of glucose gel
- 1/4 cup of orange juice (4 oz)
- 1/2 cup of regular soda (not sugar free)
- 1 Tbsp of honey or syrup
- 8 oz of nonfat (skim) milk

Glucose tablets and glucose gel are portable, so if you are at risk for hypoglycemia, you should carry them with you at all times. If you take insulin and are also taking an alpha glucosidase inihibitor (such as acarbose or miglitol), keep in mind that the inhibitor, when taken, delays the absorption of carbohydrates, so glucose tablets or gel are the recommended choice.

for safety reasons. Lower targets for hypoglycemia may be recommended in women who have diabetes and are pregnant.

Always go by the blood glucose numbers. If you are in doubt, double check the test to be sure. Symptoms are useful, but numbers are facts. Once you have treated the hypoglycemia, it is wise to check 15 minutes later to verify that the treatment resolved the issue. You should never begin (or continue) exercising until the hypoglycemia is resolved. Ideally, you will have an exercise partner who knows you have diabetes and can offer you the proper assistance should you need it.

Once you've consulted with your diabetes care team about your exercise options and any necessary safety precautions, you are ready to go. Think about all the routine things you do during the day and how you might add activity into your everyday life. A good place to start is by looking at what you do during the week that include walking and come up with different ways to increase your walking efforts.

Daily walking has been shown to reduce fat around the belly, which is typical of type 2 diabetes. As adults, we appreciate feedback or information to measure what we are doing. With regard to walking, many find that a pedometer is helpful in determining the distance

BUILD UP TO 30 MINUTES OF BRISK WALKING FIVE DAYS A WEEK

	Warm Up Time	Fast Walk Time	Cool Down Time	Total Time
WEEK 1	walk slowly 5 min.	walk briskly 5 min.	walk slowly 5 min.	15 min.
WEEK 2	walk slowly 5 min.	walk briskly 8 min.	walk slowly 5 min.	18 min.
WEEK 3	walk slowly 5 min.	walk briskly 11 min.	walk slowly 5 min.	21 min.
WEEK 4	walk slowly 5 min.	walk briskly 14 min.	walk slowly 5 min.	24 min.
WEEK 5	walk slowly 5 min.	walk briskly 17 min.	walk slowly 5 min.	27 min.
WEEK 6	walk slowly 5 min.	walk briskly 20 min.	walk slowly 5 min.	30 min.
WEEK 7	walk slowly 5 min.	walk briskly 23 min.	walk slowly 5 min.	33 min.
WEEK 8	walk slowly 5 min.	walk briskly 26 min.	walk slowly 5 min.	36 min.
WEEK 9+	walk slowly 5 min.	walk briskly 30 min.	walk slowly 5 min.	40 min.

National Diabetes Education Program, National Institutes of Health. Small Steps Big Rewards: Your Game Plan, *2003.*

walked on a daily basis. Basic models may be found for as little as $10, while high-tech versions can cost significantly more. Because pedometers sense movement, they are not good at making fine measurements. They are helpful in giving you a general idea of what you are doing. Keep in mind that movement as simple as squirming in your chair can be picked up by a pedometer. Some pedometers don't begin counting until you have taken at least five steps to ensure that the movement is repetitive. Don't worry: The pedometer will credit you if you keep moving. The best position for a pedometer is clipped to a belt or your waist directly over the crease of your pant leg. Failure to keep it level can throw off the count.

The number of steps recommended for you on a daily basis may vary depending on your age, strength, and physical health. Walking 10,000 steps is an approximate equivalent to walking five miles. If you are trying to work up to the 10,000 step recommendation, build up gradually. Keep track of the number of steps you are walking on a daily basis for one week by wearing a pedometer. At the end of the week, take the highest number of steps you walked on a given day and use that as your starting baseline. If this number is comfortable for you, add 500 steps per day the following week. Keep increasing until you reach 10,000 (or as many steps as you can tolerate). While walking outside is usually preferred, indoor alternatives like mall walking or using a treadmill are great options to help you stay on track if the weather is less than desirable.

As you are walking your way to better health, jump in and enjoy the benefits, but please make sure you are tolerating the exercise well. There are several ways to tell if you are overdoing physical activity while you are exercising. One of the ways you can evaluate how well you may be tolerating the intensity of your exercise is by doing the "talk test." The other is by using the Borg Rate of Perceived Exertion (RPE). Make an effort to try these techniques to help you evaluate your exercise intensity.

EVALUATING INTENSITY OF EXERCISE

Talk Test: An individual should be able to talk with someone while performing an activity

Borg RPE: An individual rates his or her level of exercise effort on a scale

0   1   2   3   4   5   6   7   8   9   10

"feels nothing at all"   "moderate"   "strong"   "very, very strong; maximal"

Adapted from The "I Hate to Exercise" Book, 2006.

The impact of exercise should be comfortable. Lower impact exercises are often the best choice, especially if you suffer from any long-term diabetes complications.

Another consideration is properly fitted shoes, which are essential during regular physical activity and exercise. The American Diabetes Association recommends using shoes with cushioned midsoles (gel or air) as well as polyester or blend (cotton-polyester) socks to keep feet dry and prevent blisters during exercise.

Your diabetes care team has probably recommended that you personally monitor your blood glucose values and keep a record or log book to analyze your blood glucose control (see Chapter 4). It may be helpful to add a section to your log that keeps track of your activity levels as well. By doing this, you can review your progress, keep track of any challenges you face, identify any relapse in your efforts, and record how well you enjoy the physical activity. All of this provides information as to the likelihood of continuing exercise on a long-term basis.

Comparing your blood glucose levels to your exercise efforts can give you information about the effect of exercise and physical activity on your blood glucose control. Look at the days of the week when you were more successful with physical activity efforts as compared to those days you weren't. What was different about the days? Were you busy at work when exercise seemed to falter? Was your daily pattern different? For example, were you required to sit more on days that your activity levels were lower? Focus on the days when it was more challenging for you to exercise. Think about how you can make changes to improve your pattern. Keep in mind that adding a few steps every day can go a long way toward meeting your exercise and physical activity goals.

STEPPING YOUR WAY TOWARD YOUR GOALS

What are your ideas for things you can do to increase your physical activity? Think about things that you could already be doing to add steps to your day. It is all about choices!

- Got a dog? Walk it.
- Have a flight of stairs handy? Use them.
- Want to limit TV time? Lose the remote control.
- Parking your car? Choose a space at the rear of the lot.
- Going somewhere? Walk.
- Kids practicing sports? Walk while you watch.
- Talking on the phone? Walk during the call.
- Going on a shopping spree? Walk the mall as opposed to surfing the Net.
- Loading groceries into the car? Walk the cart to the corral.

Consider the benefit of resistance exercises, including weight lifting and other strength training methods. An ideal exercise program includes both and can help you preserve strength and healthy oxygen levels in the blood for up to 20 years longer. This translates into a higher level of independence as you age. If you are a woman who is post-menopausal, resistance exercises can help preserve bone mineral density, keeping your bones stronger and less likely to fracture from osteoporosis.

The size of a muscle is affected by the amount of activity performed. As you think about improving your strength, keep the following considerations in mind:

- Warm up! Start by walking briskly, marching in place, or riding a stationary bicycle for about 5–10 minutes. Go through your routine

BUILDING STRENGTH AND ENDURANCE

- To build strength, choose a weight that you can lift only two to six times while resting for a few minutes between sets.

- To build endurance, choose a weight that you can lift 15–20 times while resting for no more than one minute between sets.

- To build both strength and endurance (combination training), choose a weight that you can lift only 8 to 12 times while resting 1–2 minutes between sets.

- Whether you use barbells or weight machines, the results are usually similar. Sit-ups, pull-ups, and push-ups are also strength building exercises in which your own body acts as the weight that you lift.

- Before you start with resistance training, consult with your diabetes care team. Consider meeting with a physical therapist, exercise physiologist, and personal trainer to make sure the program is safe and right for you.

Adapted from Roberts, SS. Secrets of Strength. Diabetes Forecast. August 2002.

slowly without weights, stretching as you do so. This helps raise your core body temperature by a couple of degrees. You can also stretch in between sets of weight training.

- Perform sets of weight resistance training that are recommended for you. Movement should be fluid, so lift and lower the weights in a slow, smooth manner.

- Breathe out when you lift weights and in when you lower weights (DO NOT hold your breath).

- Maintain an upright posture.

- Cool down by stretching for 5–10 minutes.

The American Diabetes Association and the American College of Sports Medicine recommend that you train at least twice weekly, doing 8–12 repetitions per set of 8–10 exercises targeting major muscle groups. There is no time like the present to get started. It may be helpful to start with the larger muscle groups (chest) and then move on to the smaller muscle groups (biceps). As you plan the days you will include resistance training in your exercise program, keep in mind that it is best to avoid consecutive days, allowing your muscles to heal in between sessions. Always try and let a day pass before your next training occurs.

How are you doing with walking? Is it an enjoyable and effective method of physical activity for you? Are you building up to 30 minutes five days a week? Building up gradually and safely is the key.

You want to make sure your feet are tolerating your exercise and physical activity. Check your feet daily for blisters, sores, itching, callus formation, or any other injuries. If you have neuropathy (damage to the nerves where feeling and sensation is altered) in your feet, your diabetes care team may recommend an alternate form of exercise for you to avoid the risk of injuring your feet.

Taking the pressure off your feet, if necessary, may involve the use of some alternative exercises that can be done sitting in a chair. Use a sturdy chair, preferably one without arms. You will want the chair to be wide enough and the back tall enough to provide your body with support. Your feet should rest squarely on the floor. Consult with a specialist in this area to determine the best options for this type of exercise. As with all exercise, this program should include a warmup phase before the activity and a cool down phase at the end.

Be sure to consult with your diabetes care team on the benefits versus the risks of any exercise program. Keep in mind: Where there is a will, there is a way.

Sometimes it is easier to get motivated than it is to stay motivated. While there is no concrete solution to guarantee you will stay motivated to perform your exercise and physical activity efforts for the rest of your life, you are the one responsible when it comes to you!

Make a commitment to keep exercise and physical activity efforts going—in writing. By making a written statement that outlines your commitment, you are telling yourself that this is serious. It may be helpful to make the commitment with family or friends present, those who can hold you accountable (without making you feel guilty). Things to include in the written statement might be your specific goals, the amount of activity and duration of time you will work on the goals, and any reward system (something like new clothes rather than food).

Focus on what you are doing (not what you aren't doing). Make a weekly summary of your accomplishments. You may find that your activity log is helpful in determining the good things you are doing.

WALK FOR A CAUSE

Step Out to Fight Diabetes, formerly America's Walk for Diabetes, is about changing the face of diabetes in our country—by raising funds to help find a cure and by walking a few miles to bring a greater awareness to this devastating disease.

Diabetes is the fastest growing disease in the United States, and Step Out's purpose is to raise funds to find a cure. This annual fundraiser kicks off in 200 cities throughout the U.S., so wherever you are, gather your friends and family and walk toward a cure. Together, we can crush this epidemic.

To register for the walk or request more information, visit the American Diabetes Association website at www.diabetes.org/stepout, or call your local American Diabetes Association office at 1-888-DIABETES.

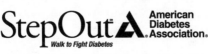

If you find it difficult, ask an objective party to help you. Sometimes those around us see things we don't see.

Plan for the unexpected. No matter how well you plan, life can change on a whim. As your routine changes, think about what you did to be successful before and use these trouble-shooting strategies to help you incorporate being active into your current schedule. Anything you can do to add some extra activity into your day is ultimately worth it.

Remember you are human and you aren't perfect. Please take the time to recognize all of the positive changes you have made—maybe even make a list of those positive changes to recognize your accomplishments. Next, make note of what you have learned from the experience.

How has your physical activity and exercise changed since week number one? Are you making a conscious decision to add more walking into your day? How many steps are you up to? What can you do to add steps as you move forward with your plan?

How will you know if your physical activity and exercise changes have made a difference in your diabetes control? Ask yourself the following…

EXERCISE HELPS TO BURN UP CALORIES

Forms of Aerobic Exercise	Calories Burned in 30 min.*
Aerobic dance/group dance	205
Dance, general (e.g., ballroom)	153
Bicycling/cycling (leisurely)	136
Hiking	204
Jogging/running	239
Rope skipping	341
Skating	239
Swimming	273
Water exercise	136
Walking	119

*Determinations are for moderate activity for an individual who weighs 150 pounds.

Adapted from Ainsworth, BA, Haskell, WL, Leon, AS, et al. Compendium of Physical Activities: Classification of Energy Costs of Human Physical Activities. Medical Science Sports Exercise. 1993; 25: 71–80.

- Do you feel better?

- How do you feel about yourself?

- Are you tolerating exercise and physical activity that is comfortable for you?

- What is your A1C?

You can determine the effect of physical activity on your blood glucose control by monitoring before and after exercise (it is usually most helpful to do both to compare the difference). Keep in mind that exercise and physical activity can have a domino effect, causing your body to be more sensitive to insulin for several hours after exercising.

Maintain a good attitude with regard to exercise and physical activity. Variety is the spice of life, so if you get bored with a particular activity, you can always make a change. Think about making your exercise activities a family affair, because if you think about it your blood relatives are at risk for type 2 diabetes. After all, no one is too young or too old to build activity into their lives.

CHAPTER 4 | Monitoring—Don't Give Up on Excellence

In any given individual, blood glucose levels will vary throughout the day, rising after a meal and returning to normal within two hours after eating. Blood glucose levels in the adult population are normally between 65 and 99 mg/dL in the morning after an overnight fast. Fasting implies going all night—or at the very least eight hours—without eating or drinking. It is generally acceptable for blood glucose levels to rise within the two hour time period after one starts eating foods or drinking liquids containing sugar or other carbohydrates, as long as the blood glucose level stays lower than 140 mg/dL.

As a person ages, normal levels will increase slightly but progressively after age 50, especially in those who lead sedentary lifestyles. For the blood glucose to stay within normal range, the body relies on the release of insulin. If insulin is working as it should, blood glucose levels will stay within normal range.

Your Blood Glucose

Regardless of the type of diabetes you have, controlling blood glucose levels is important for your diabetes health. Both short term, to

NORMAL VS. ABNORMAL BLOOD GLUCOSE

Normal Blood Glucose	Impaired Blood Glucose	Elevated Blood Glucose**
Fasting 65–99 mg/dL*	Fasting: 100–125 mg/dL	Fasting: 126 mg/dL
	Casual: 140–199 mg/dL[†]	Casual: >200 mg/dL[†]

*should stay <140mg/dL after meals

**2 values exceeding these values on random occasions indicate a diagnosis of diabetes

[†] "casual" blood glucose is without regard to fasting

Adapted from: American Diabetes Association. Clinical Practice Recommendation: Standards of Medical Care. Diabetes Care 31:S13, January 2008.

help you feel better on a day-to-day basis, and long term, by keeping blood glucose within ranges so your risk for complications is lower.

If you have diabetes, keeping your blood glucose controlled is not at all a simple task. In fact, it takes a whole lot of work and commitment. Data suggest that the more you monitor your blood glucose levels when you have diabetes, the better control you have. Why is that? It is not because monitoring automatically translates into perfect blood glucose levels, but rather because it provides you with information to make the best decisions to help you make timely improvements in your diabetes treatment plan for optimal blood glucose control.

Routinely checking your blood glucose level provides you and your diabetes care team with information to help you customize your treatment plan to best benefit your diabetes control. Blood glucose levels are either within recommended ranges, higher than recommended, or, in some cases, too low. Once you know where you are with respect to your blood glucose levels, you can take the necessary action for improvement.

Healthy adults with diabetes should work toward the best possible blood glucose control. Recommended goals are based on proven research that optimal blood glucose control does reduce your risk for the complications to the nerves and blood vessels that occur from high blood glucose levels.

ADA TARGETS FOR BLOOD GLUCOSE IN HEALTHY ADULTS WITH DIABETES

Fasting and preprandial (pre-meal): 70–130 mg/dL

Postprandial (1–2 hours after a meal): <180 mg/dL (at peak)

A1C: <7.0%*

*The A1C target for the individual person with diabetes is an A1C as close to normal (<6%) as possible without significant hypoglycemia.

Adapted from: American Diabetes Association. Clinical Practice Recommendation: Standards of Medical Care. Diabetes Care 31:S18, January 2008.

Keep in mind that your blood glucose numbers are an investment in your health, again both short term and long term. One example that might be helpful is to think about purchasing stock options. When you buy or invest in a stock, you don't just close your eyes and pick one out. You think about the investment as one that will improve over time. But whatever you do, you don't ignore it. Based on the numbers and analysis, you make decisions on buying or selling. Your blood glucose levels are similar. You monitor the numbers so that if they aren't satisfactory, you can make changes by working with your diabetes care team and troubleshooting the numbers with the goal of improvement. You watch your overall control (blood glucose records and patterns) to see how you are doing. Whatever you do, don't ignore your blood glucose control, even if you don't feel bad—because you will lose, and your risk for long-term complications will go up.

If you have been monitoring your blood glucose levels, that is great! If you haven't, there is no time like the present to get started. It is always a good idea to make sure your blood glucose meter is in working order and your test strips are up to date. If your strips are un-opened, they are good until the manufacturer expiration date stamped on the bottle (or box). If they have been opened, then they are good for a much shorter time period, usually 2–3 months. It is a good idea to check the test strip insert from the company to verify how long the strips are recommended for use once opened. Using the opened test strips outside the recommended range can lead to inaccurate results when testing your blood.

If your meter is more than a couple of years old, ask your diabetes care team about an update. Many times they will have sample meters that are the newer versions that you can use to obtain your routine blood glucose checks. You can also call the company that manufactures your meter to see what options are currently available. Many times, the company will upgrade your meter to the newest and most efficient product. Keep in mind that access to the appropriate supplies may be better with updated versions of self-monitoring equipment. If you have insurance, you should inquire about the coverage you have for an updated model. You will probably need a prescription for the blood glucose monitor and supplies to obtain insurance coverage for these necessary items.

Each meter company has a toll-free number listed on the back of the particular meter. If you aren't sure about the meter you have and how reliable it is, you can obtain a glucose control solution that is made for the meter, which most pharmacies carry. The glucose control solution can be used to verify that the meter and testing supplies are in working order. To perform a test, shake the bottle and apply a drop of solution to the test strip (as recommended by the manufacturer's user guide). The solution on the strip is then read by the meter similar to a blood glucose sample. The solution contains a controlled amount of glucose that, when applied correctly, should read within a certain designated range printed on the test strip packaging. You should check to make sure that the control solution has not passed the expiration date that is printed on the bottle or the discard date, which is usually the date opened plus about three months. If the result of your control solution test does not read within the specified range, you may want to repeat it to verify. If it is still not within the recommended range, use the toll-free number located on the back of the meter to contact the meter company. It is a good idea to check your blood glucose meter with glucose control solution at least once a year.

Assuring that your meter is in the best possible working order is essential so that you can rely on the results you obtain to help you maximize your efforts in improving your blood glucose control.

The information that you gather from self-monitoring of blood glucose should be useful to you and your diabetes care team. Consult with your diabetes care team to determine the times of day that you should monitor. Common times that are recommended include, fasting (pre-breakfast), before lunch, before supper, and before bedtime.

Before meals

Pre-meal blood glucose checks are probably the most commonly recommended checks. This includes before each meal, with the pre-breakfast check most likely being your fasting check (after 8–12 hours of no food intake), first thing after waking up. Pre-meal checks provide information about your overall diabetes treatment plan.

After meals

Your diabetes care team might recommend checking approximately 1 to 2 hours after you begin eating. This result is probably most useful if you check before the meal, and compare that with the post-meal result. The after meal value can assist you and your diabetes care team to evaluate the effect of diabetes medications that are taken with the intent of controlling post meal blood glucose. These numbers may also assist you in determining the effect of carbohydrate intake from your meals, helping you make decisions about the impact of the amount and the type of carbohydrate you are eating. If you have pre-meal blood glucose values within your target ranges, yet your A1C remains above target, then monitoring post-meal values with diabetes care intervention(s) to reduce post-meal blood glucose to meet recommended goals may improve your A1C. There may be an advantage in post-meal glucose control to cardiovascular health. Some epidemiological studies have associated elevated post-challenge (2-hour oral glucose tolerance test) glucose values with increased cardiovascular risk independent of fasting plasma glucose.

Bedtime

Occasional bedtime checks may be recommended to determine if your blood glucose level is safe for you prior to going to bed. Bedtime checks compared to fasting blood glucose checks (the next morning) can verify the effects of your treatment plan and how it works overnight. They may help you to determine the need for a bedtime snack prior to retiring for the night.

Middle of the night

Checking your blood glucose level in the middle of the night is particularly useful to *insulin users* to determine if blood glucose levels are maintained at a reasonably safe level during the night. Your diabetes care team will usually recommend that a middle of the night reading be taken sometime between 2 and 4 a.m. This is especially true for those taking intermediate or long-acting insulin therapy injected at supper or bedtime, as well as in evaluating pre-programmed overnight basal rates if you are using an insulin pump. In some cases, if fasting or pre-breakfast levels are too high, it can be the result of rebounding from glucose levels that have dropped too low during the night.

Other common times

It is important to check your blood glucose level with feelings of hyperglycemia and hypoglycemia to verify the feelings and symptoms. If your blood glucose level is too high or too low, following up promptly to remedy the situation is key. It is important to establish with your diabetes care team a plan ahead of time to treat these hyperglycemia or hypoglycemia events. Blood glucose monitoring can also be beneficial in assisting you to evaluate the effects of exercise and physical activity on blood glucose control. In addition, it is important to check your blood glucose before driving or operating machinery to avoid any situations that could become dangerous if hypoglycemia should occur. You can also check your blood glucose levels whenever you feel necessary.

It is important to keep a record of your blood glucose levels. Be sure and take the record with you when you visit your health care providers. This usually begins with you writing down your blood glucose levels. You will want to make sure to include the day and time, blood glucose result, any medication taken and any adjustments made, as well as what you ate and any exercise you participated in. Many meters have the option of downloading the results with company-based software. To find out more about this option, ask your diabetes care team or call the toll-free number on the back of your meter. Regardless of the method you choose for tracking your blood glucose results, the important thing is that you have information to review to help you and your diabetes team make decisions about your care.

KEEPING TRACK OF MY BLOOD GLUCOSE NUMBERS*

Using a record log book can help you determine patterns and whether or not your are meeting your goals.

Daily Diabetes Record   Week Starting _____

	Mon	Tues	Wed	Thurs	Fri	Sat	Sun
Other Blood Glucose							
Breakfast Blood Glucose	156 mg/dL			139 mg/dL			154 mg/dL
Medicine							
Lunch Blood Glucose		185 mg/dL			155 mg/dL		
Medicine							
Dinner Blood Glucose			90 mg/dL			85 mg/dL	
Medicine							
Bedtime Blood Glucose							
Medicine							
Notes (Special events, sick days, exercise)							

This is an example only and in no way reflects personal goals.

General recommendations on how often you should check your blood glucose levels will likely depend on the type of diabetes you have, your treatment plan, recommendations by your diabetes care team, and your insurance coverage for monitoring supplies. Insulin users, especially those who take several injections a day, should monitor their blood glucose at least three or more times daily. Those with type 2 diabetes, who use insulin less frequently, use other diabetes medications, or manage their diabetes without the use of medications (meal planning and physical activity alone), should monitor their blood glucose as recommended by their diabetes care team. No matter what your treatment plan, you should monitor your blood glucose levels frequently to see if your diabetes management plan is working.

The key is to make the most out of the strip coverage you have. If you are paying on your own, then you may have to adjust your routine for blood glucose checks according to your budget. Work with your diabetes care team to optimize your monitoring schedule. Always rely on your blood glucose numbers as opposed to symptoms. While paying attention to your symptoms is helpful to overall blood glucose control, monitoring is the best way to make sure you are staying within the desired range and will help to optimize your overall health.

Congratulations! It is great that you are checking your blood glucose levels on a routine basis. It is also important that you collaborate with your diabetes care team to monitor your progress. Questions you may want to think about are:

- Is my blood glucose control improving?

- If so, is my overall control based on various checks throughout the day improving?

- Are there any problem areas?

- If there are problem areas, what might be a possible solution?

- Can I improve blood glucose at a certain time of day without upsetting progress at other times of the day?

- Am I closely monitoring when my routine changes (meal plan, usual exercise and physical activities, or if I begin feeling ill)?

Once you visit your diabetes care team, you should always set a plan to follow through with reporting your blood glucose results, especially when you make changes to your treatment plan. The only way that you and your diabetes care team are going to know if what you are doing is working is to collaborate on your results. Check with your team to see what method (i.e., drop off, fax, email, or download) is preferred for you to get your records to them.

Additional adjustments to your treatment plan can be made based on your blood glucose values. Don't wait: Focus on timely communication with your diabetes care team to make sure any adjustments made meet the goal of making your treatment plan as individualized as possible. Some people have an aversion to sticking their fingers and producing a blood sample to check their blood glucose levels. While fingertips have traditionally been used for sampling blood glucose, some meters work with blood samples from other sites, including the arm, thigh, or calf. If alternative site testing is important to you, be sure that the meter you have, or one that you might purchase, is approved for alternative site testing. Also, find out which alternative sites you can use with it.

Not all meters are approved for the same sites and some sites may not be right for you. These meters can usually be used with the fingertips in addition to the alternative site. Be sure you are instructed in the proper use of the meter, because the procedure and equipment may be different when sticking the alternative site as opposed to the fingertips. It is generally best to use the fingertips when rapid blood glucose changes are likely to occur—when you have recently exercised or taken insulin or if you have eaten within the last two hours. Blood flow reaches the finger or palm at the base of the thumb 3–5 times faster than alternate sites. Fingertip samples may show these changes sooner than other areas. It is best to discuss with your diabetes care team whether alternative site testing is right for you.

Just checking your blood glucose levels is not enough. Those numbers are yours and if they aren't meeting the goals you and your diabetes care team have set, review the results and figure out when you need to work on them. It is important to have a record of your blood glucose levels that you and your diabetes care team can analyze. You will want to make sure that the record allows you to see the patterns of your blood glucose numbers. If you have been writing your blood glucose levels down, that is a good start; however, keep in mind that looking at the patterns is key to making any necessary changes to your plan.

DAILY BLOOD GLUCOSE RECORD*

For example, let's say you have been checking once daily for the past week and a half. You are recording your blood glucose levels down the page on a legal pad. So, your record looks like this:

Monday at 7 a.m—156 mg/dl

Tuesday at 11:30 a.m.—185 mg/dl

Wednesday at 6:30 p.m.—90 mg/dl

Thursday at 7:10 a.m.—139 mg/dl

Friday at 12:30 p.m.—155 mg/dl

Saturday at 8:00 p.m.—85 mg/dl

Sunday at 9 a.m. —154 mg/dl

Monday at 11:30 a.m.—199 mg/dl

Tuesday at 7:00 a.m.—110 mg/dl

Wednesday at 7:00 a.m.—144mg/dl

*This is an example only and in no way reflects personal goals.

Many praises for your efforts; however, it is difficult to review and figure out any patterns to this list of blood glucose values. It is also difficult to scroll through the meter memory and detect patterns.

If you are relying on the meter memory, it is best if you go back 1–2 weeks to retrieve results and record them. Make sure your meter clock (date and time) are set correctly so the information you are recording reflects the date and time that the results actually occurred. You may prefer downloading your blood glucose results. Many meter companies have programs and software that can be purchased to provide you with an electronic record that can be printed. Most of the programs can be customized so that they best meet your needs.

Your action plan for diabetes care will include a goal for the best possible blood glucose control for you. As you continue to monitor your blood glucose levels, how are they doing from your perspective? When you review your records, do you see the blood glucose levels meeting the goals that you and your diabetes care team have set?

For those blood glucose levels that you are happy with, continue checking to keep them within goal. For those that are not, think about other information that you might need to help you analyze the values on a deeper level. You are keeping track of the date, time, and test result. Think about other information that may provide clues, such as:

• Timing and types of diabetes medication you are taking

• What and how much you ate (tracking total number of carbohydrates eaten)

• Activity levels throughout the day (time, frequency, and intensity)

Be as detailed as possible; this information may be particularly useful as you fine-tune your blood glucose numbers. As you continue your life journey with diabetes, you may want to pick a week each month to keep more detailed records to help you keep a close check on how you are doing. If your blood glucose levels start to creep up, it might be a good idea to keep 1–2 weeks of detailed records to see what factors are contributing to it. Your diabetes care team may recommend that you monitor more frequently under certain situations that may alter your blood glucose control.

MORE FREQUENT BLOOD GLUCOSE CHECKS: MONITOR THESE SITUATIONS

Keeping a close eye on your blood glucose levels is always important; however, the following situations require more frequent checks:

- If you are unable to verbalize or recognize symptoms of hypoglycemia
- If you are experiencing a period of stress to the body—illness, infection, surgery, or pregnancy
- If you have had a recent change in medications that alter blood glucose control
- If you have added a new medication that influences blood glucose levels (i.e., steroid therapy)
- If you have noticed an increase in hypoglycemic events
- If you have experienced unexplained changes in your weight
- If you have noticed deterioration in your diabetes control
- If you have made changes in your diabetes treatment plan, such as increase or decrease in calories or activity levels

Keep in mind that as you age with diabetes, it is normal for your body to change, which may require a change in your treatment plan. Staying in touch with regard to your body and blood glucose control will help support making necessary changes in a timely manner to avoid sacrificing your diabetes control.

Adapted from Joslin EZ Start™ Monitoring Schedules and Frequency. 3.4 SMBG and Glycemic Goals, 2006.

As you review your blood glucose levels, think about any differences you see from one day to the next. For example, if you were more active on Monday, Wednesday, and Friday versus Tuesday and Thursday, how did that affect your overall blood glucose levels? If Tuesday and Thursday are typically more sedentary days, what can you do to add activity on those days?

It's also a good idea to do a quick carbohydrate check on days your blood glucose levels are higher, particularly if elevated after meals. Keeping track of total carbohydrate intake is helpful to assure you are getting the targeted amounts. As good as you are at counting those carbs, food labels can be misread or portions can be miscalculated. Don't fret if that happens to you, just chalk it up as a learning experience and maybe take some time to brush up on your skill. Check in with your diabetes care team regarding how your control is doing, what ideas you have about it, and any theories you have for making changes.

Just a reminder that no one is perfect—not you or the health care professionals who take care of you. Anything you do toward improving your blood glucose control makes a difference in your diabetes health. Pat yourself on the back for the time and effort you have put in. You are genuinely worth it!

Your A1C level should be checked routinely by your diabetes care team. In most individuals with diabetes, it is done about every 3–4 months. If your diabetes control is stable, your physician may perform the test every six months. You can always ask to have an A1C performed to determine how well your overall blood glucose control is doing, as well as provide you with information to help you determine your risk for the long-term complications of diabetes.

The closer your A1C is to normal, the lower your risk for the complications of diabetes—eye disease (retinopathy), kidney disease (nephropathy), and nerve damage (neuropathy). For every percentage point that you reduce your A1C, you lower your risk for complications from diabetes. The American Diabetes Association recommends an A1C of less than 7%, or an A1C as close to normal (<6%) as possible without significant hypoglycemia.

If you have been monitoring your blood glucose levels and are seeing an improvement, asking for an A1C is great validation that your control is improving. A1C is glucose attached to hemoglobin, a protein found in red blood cells that move oxygen from your lungs to other parts of your body. A1C is the part of the hemoglobin that has been glycosolated (or has added glucose). Since an average red blood cell lives about 120 days, the A1C is an average of glucose attached to the red blood cells for that period of time. Because blood glucose levels in the preceding 30 days contribute more to the A1C than the 90–120 days earlier, 30–60 days of improved blood glucose control can contribute significantly to a drop in the A1C.

Keep in mind that the A1C detects the amount of glucose attached to normal hemoglobin. The following can keep your A1C test from producing valid results.

• If you have a hemoglobin variant, such as sickle-cell anemia or some forms of thalassemia (a group of inherited disorders resulting from an imbalance in hemoglobin production), your A1C test may not be valid. Because of these abnormalities, the test could measure lower even if your blood glucose has been running high.

- Some drugs can interfere with the A1C reading. High aspirin doses can contribute to higher than expected A1C levels.

- If you have a build-up of a product called urea in your bloodstream—which is common in kidney disease—your A1C test may also show a false high.

- If your red blood cells don't live the expected lifespan (approximately 120 days), then your A1C may be falsely low. This can be the result of certain disease states or even genetic factors.

- If you have had a recent blood transfusion, red blood cells may falsely affect your A1C.

As with any laboratory test, there are some limitations to the A1C; however, it is a very useful tool to assist with monitoring diabetes control. You as the consumer with diabetes need to know your A1C. Each 1% change in A1C equals the equivalent of approximately a 35 mg/dL change in blood glucose. So, if you want to see how far you've come with behavior change and improvement in blood glucose control, ask your diabetes care team to measure your A1C!

A1C TARGETS FOR HEALTHY (NON-PREGNANT) ADULTS WITH DIABETES

The A1C test gives a snapshot of blood glucose control over the previous 2–3 months. The lower your A1C, the better your chances are of avoiding serious diabetes complications. Check to see how A1C test results translate to an average blood glucose value:

A1C test result	6%	7%	8%	9%	10%	11%	12%
Average plasma glucose level	135 mg/dL	170 mg/dL	205 mg/dL	240 mg/dL	275 mg/dL	310 mg/dL	345 mg/dL

A1C targets may be modified in certain adult populations, such as women who are pregnant (typically lower) and the elderly (sometimes higher).

Adapted from: American Diabetes Association. Clinical Practice Recommendation: Standards of Medical Care. Diabetes Care 31:S18, January 2008.

MONITORING—DON'T
GIVE UP ON EXCELLENCE

CHAPTER 5

Taking Medication— Is It Necessary?

When meal planning and exercise are not enough to control your blood glucose levels, you will need to take medications to maintain optimum blood glucose control and health. Your health care provider will prescribe the medications to control your blood glucose, lipids, and blood pressure. Adding medications to your treatment plan does not mean you have failed. It doesn't mean your diabetes has become worse. It only means that your previous treatment plan is no longer working to adequately control your blood glucose levels.

Expect that your treatment plan will change over time. Why does it have to change? One reason is the natural progression of type 2 diabetes. In the beginning, your body slowly loses the ability to react to glucose rapidly entering the body when eating a meal. When insulin secretion cannot keep up with a post-meal rise in glucose, it is called the first phase loss of insulin secretion. You might notice normal fasting blood glucose or higher than normal blood glucose two hours after a meal. As time progresses, the body will have difficulty managing the background insulin or basal insulin secretion that maintains your fasting blood glucose level. This is the second phase loss of insulin secretion and you will see elevated or abnormal fasting blood glucose levels. As you change, so will the medications used to control your diabetes.

The development of new and improved drugs and techniques for delivering medications every year may have an effect on your medication dosages. Your diabetes management plan should be dynamic, changing with your needs and the availability of new technology, medications, and research.

The goal of therapy is to develop a medication plan that will closely mimic the normal release of insulin from the pancreas to provide background and mealtime insulin, maintaining optimum glucose control. Everyone is different and medications are recommended based on you as an individual. One medication will not be effective for everyone with diabetes. Luckily, there are many choices and combinations of therapy.

Types of Medications

Medications for diabetes are found in two major groups: oral agents and injectables. Oral agents are pills that help you control your blood glucose levels, and are specifically used to treat type 2 diabetes. Type 2 diabetes involves several underlying problems with the way sources of energy are processed by the body; therefore, there may be a number of possible medication solutions.

QUESTIONS TO ASK YOUR DIABETES CARE TEAM

For your diabetes medication management plan, ask:

- What do I do if I miss a dose? (it is usually best not to double up on the next dose)
- Should I take this medication with food or water?
- Is there anything to avoid when starting this medication (driving, operating heavy machinery, etc.)?
- What if I have side effect such as rash or stomach problems?

Keeping a record is usually the best way to identify concerns and possible issues that might occur with your diabetes medication plan.

Oral agents

There are six classes of oral medications for type 2 diabetes:

- *Alpha-glucosidase inhibitors.* The major site of action is in the intestines. The alpha-glucosidase inhibitor slows down the rate at which the intestine breaks down food into glucose. This causes glucose to enter your blood more slowly; therefore, glucose remains at a consistent level, resulting in fewer highs and lows. The end result is flattening out elevations in glucose that may occur after meals.

- *Biguanides*. The major site of action is in the liver. The biguanide slowly lowers the amount of stored glucose that is released from your liver into your body. It increases the sensitivity of the body cells to insulin, allowing more glucose into the cells. These actions keep blood glucose levels consistent.

- *DPP-4 inhibitors*. The major site of action is in the gut. They help the body by blocking an enzyme that inactivates the natural hormones in the body called Glucagon-like Peptide (GLP-1) and glucose-dependent insulinotropic polypeptide (GIP). GLP-1 levels are lower in Type 2 diabetes. GLP-1 can help promote insulin production by the pancreas and inhibit glucose production by the liver. When used alone or with other oral agents that do not cause hypoclycemia, the risk for low blood glucose reactions is low. DPP-4 will usually not cause weight gain.

- *Meglitinides and D-phenylalanine derivatives*. The major site of action is in the pancreas. They cause the pancreas to secrete more insulin. Although not sulfonylureas, they work in a similar fashion. They are taken before meals and produce insulin for a short period of time to cover post-meal elevations. Low blood glucose reactions can occur, but the risk is lower than with a sulfonylurea.

- *Sulfonylureas*. The major site of action is in the pancreas. They help the body secrete more insulin, thus lowering blood glucose levels. Sulfonylureas can cause low blood glucose reactions. Over time, these medications may no longer control blood glucose, causing levels to rise.

- *Thiazolidinediones*. The major site of action is in muscle. They lower your body's resistance to insulin at the cellular level of muscle and fat. Thiazolidinediones reverse insulin resistance by making the cells more receptive to insulin, allowing more glucose to enter the cells where it is used as energy. This action results in lower blood glucose levels.

At some point in your therapy, your health care provider may prescribe a combination oral agent. Although not a class of oral agents, combination pills are widely used. Combination pills contain two classes of oral agents in one pill. This medication can target two different defects that cause elevated blood glucose in type 2 diabetes. Combination therapy offers several benefits, including improved blood glucose control over a single agent, ease of administration, and improved adherence because it is simpler to take one pill than two.

Injectable medications

Insulin

People with type 1 diabetes will always require insulin, and many of those with type 2 may eventually need insulin to control blood glucose levels. Insulin is a protein easily digested like the food we eat; therefore, it cannot be taken in pill form and must be either injected or, for some patients, inhaled. Treatment regimens for insulin are used to closely mimic normal insulin release from the pancreas and maintain pre-meal glucose of 130 mg/dL or lower and an A1C of less than 7% (see Chapter 4).

Premixed insulin is an option for those who want convenience or who have difficultly mixing intermediate and regular or rapid-acting insulin in one syringe. Premixed insulin is also available in a prefilled insulin pen. Pens are portable, convenient, and

TYPES OF INSULIN

Insulin is characterized by the onset of action, peak action time, and duration. Based on these characteristics there are four types of insulin:

- Rapid-acting insulin begins to work about 15 minutes or less after injection, peaking in about an hour, and works for 2–3 hours.

- Regular or short-acting insulin begins about 30 minutes after injection, peaking in about 2–3 hours, and works for 3–6 hours.

- Intermediate-acting insulin begins about 2–4 hours after injection, peaking in 4–12 hours, and works for 12–18 hours.

- Long-acting insulin begins about 2–4 hours after injection; it is generally considered "peakless," mimicking background insulin; and it lasts up to 24 hours.

easy to use. Pens are being used more widely, replacing the traditional vial and syringe. The mixtures come in human and analog insulin.

Human (recombinant DNA) insulin can be produced in large quantities. It is essentially the exact molecule that is produced by the human pancreas. Human insulin has several advantages over the beef and pork versions that were first used to treat diabetes. Analog insulin is also produced in factories in large quantities. Analog insulin acts like human insulin, but has a different chemical structure. Analog insulin has been designed with its own characteristic onset times, peak times, and duration in order to help maintain glucose control.

Other injectables

Two other injectable medications for the treatment of diabetes that were approved in 2005 are exenatide and pramlintide.

- *Exenatide.* Used to improved blood glucose in patients with type 2 diabetes. It is used with metformin, sulfonylureas, or thiazolidinediones, or in combinations of metformin and sulfonylureas or metformin and thiazolidinedione. Exenatide controls blood glucose by mimicking a naturally occuring hormone in the body called GLP-1. It works by signaling the pancreas to produce insulin, stopping the liver from releasing glucose when the body does not need it, and decreasing food intake by causing a sense of fullness when eating. It is available in a pre-filled pen and can be given by injection up to 60 minutes prior to eating the two major meals of the day, which should be at least 6 hours apart.

- *Pramlintide acetate.* A medication for people with type 1 or 2 diabetes who take mealtime insulin. It is a synthetic analog of Amylin, a naturally occuring hormone that is produced by the pancreas. This hormone is typically deficient in those people that are also insulin deficient. Pramlintide is taken within 15 minutes prior to a meal and cannot be mixed with pre-meal insulin. Pramlintide can be injected using a vial and syringe or a prefilled pen device and is helpful in controlling post-meal glucose elevations.

Insulin delivery devices

There are a number of insulin delivery devices including vials and syringes, prefilled pens, and insulin pumps or pods. Syringes have become smaller and needles shorter with finer points over time. Improvements in these devices have made injecting easier and almost pain free. Prefilled pens are easy to use, look like a large ink pen, have a lower/less clinical profile than carrying a vial and a syringe, and are convenient when away from home.

Insulin pumps provide a continuous system of insulin delivery, which helps achieve better blood glucose control. Pumps are computerized devices that deliver insulin in a continuous basal dose and a bolus dose at mealtimes. Insulin infuses from a device the size of a small cell phone through flexible plastic tubing called a catheter. Insulin pumps and pods use only rapid-acting insulin. Another system that is available is a small, lightweight, self-adhesive insulin pod that you wear on your body for up to three days. This system delivers precise, personalized doses of insulin into your body through a small flexible tube based on instructions that you program into its wireless companion. Users must be willing to check their blood glucose frequently.

Combination therapy

It is very common to see combinations of diabetes medications used because they work together to better control your blood glucose. Many people use various combinations of oral agents, insulin or other injectable drugs. Physicians prescribe combinations of diabetes medications to correct the underlying reasons for the elevated blood glucose in type 2 diabetes. These include:

- Pancreas does not produce enough insulin

- Muscle cells do not accept glucose

- Liver releases glucose inappropriately

You can see that there is a wide variety of medications to meet your individual needs to control blood glucose. They are convenient to use and will simplify your lifestyle. No matter what concerns you have, there are many options to help you succeed in controlling your blood glucose levels. There are devices that make it easier to see your syringe or pens to inject if dexterity is a problem. There are many methods to overcome needle phobis, as well as solutions if you frequently forget to take your medications.

When you think about your medications, there are three important areas on which to focus: taking medications as prescribed, taking the correct amount of the medication, and taking medications at the right time. These are critical to your optimal health. You are ultimately in control of taking your medications. The next eight weeks will add to your diabetes management plan by clarifying what you know, help you ask questions to increase your knowledge, and help set achievable goals that will improve the way you feel on a daily basis.

Taking your medications is a commitment you make to stay healthy and prevent or delay the long-term complications and avoid the short-term complications of diabetes. When you have diabetes, chances are you already have a full medicine cabinet. You may take pills for diabetes, blood pressure, and cholesterol, along with a number of over-the-counter drugs or supplements.

Taking a variety of medications means more health benefits as well as potential risks, but there are steps you can take to increase the benefits and keep the risks at a minimum. Once you commit to focusing on your medications, it will take some organization and time. Begin your organization by gathering all of your prescription and nonprescription medications.

After you have gathered all of your medications, your first step will be to make an up-to-date list of all the medications you are taking. If you obtain your medications from one pharmacy, the pharmacist should be able to print a complete list of all your prescriptions. Create a chart with the name of the medication, the dosage, the reason you are taking the medication, and the time of day you take it.

MEDICATION QUESTIONS TO ASK YOURSELF

Ask yourself these simple questions:

- What is the name of this medication?
- Why am I taking the medication?
- How much should I take?
- What time of day should I take the medication?
- How should I take the medication (with or without food)?
- How often do I use this medication?
- What problems do I have taking the medication?
- What is the expiration date?
- How many refills do I have left?

If you cannot answer these questions, find out the answers. Write down all of your questions and have them ready for your next visit to your health care provider or pharmacist.

TAKING MEDICATION—
IS IT NECESSARY?

If you already have a list of all of your medications, you're in great shape. Make sure your list is current. This is an exercise that should be done at least once every year. It can serve as the "spring cleaning" for your medicine cabinet. Be sure to dispose of expired medications, medications that have been discontinued, or drugs you no longer use.

Another valuable source of information for your questions is the insert found packaged in your medications and on labels. Always read the labels and the package inserts that come with your prescriptions. Your pharmacy may provide drug information on printed forms when you pick up your prescriptions. These sources contain important information and answers to many questions you may have. Keep the medication inserts for future reference. It is estimated that 50% of people do not take their prescriptions correctly, causing drugs to work less effectively. It becomes a greater issue if you take many different medications either prescribed or not prescribed. Don't forget to read the labels on your over-the-counter vitamins, pain relievers, heartburn medications, cold medicines, allergy medications, and herbal supplements as well. All of these can cause side effects if taken improperly.

Write down any questions you have and obtain answers. Make copies of your medication record to share with your diabetes health care team at doctor appointments. Everyone is nervous at their health appointments and stress can interfere with your memory. Having the list with you makes it easier to recall the medications you are taking, particularly if you are meeting with several different health care providers. To achieve better blood glucose control, it is important to manage your medications. Maintaining a file with your medical records, medication record, medication inserts, and pharmacy information on each of the medications you take is a great start to maximizing your diabetes control.

According to a study by the National Electronic Injury Surveillance System, emergency room visits due to adverse events related to diabetes pills account for 14,500 emergency room visits every year. The number is far greater if you consider those people who were seen in clinics, doctors' offices, or treated over the phone. Most adverse events are related to mistakenly taking a second dose, thus doubling up on a medication.

Some medications for type 2 diabetes can cause side effects or interactions with other medications. Using one pharmacy for all your prescriptions can help you avoid medication errors by decreasing the chance of taking the same medication twice by mistake or preventing interactions that sometimes occur when some medications are taken together. The pharmacy can also alert you if a medication has been ordered that may cause an allergic reaction.

One of the most common side effects of medications that increase insulin in the bloodstream—such as sulfonylureas or injecting insulin—is the risk of hypoglycemia. You may experience hypoglycemia if lifestyle factors like exercise or food intake are out of balance with your medications. Treatment of hypoglycemia is easily treated with 15 grams of fast-acting carbohydrates, which should start working in about 20 minutes. Medications like biguanides do not have a risk for hypoglycemia because insulin sensitizers work at the cellular level. It is important to understand how each of your medications works in the body to determine if you are at risk for hypoglycemia.

Some studies have shown that people with diabetes are taking as many as 4–5 different medications at a time. Medications taken to reduce high blood pressure will raise blood glucose levels. If you take blood pressure medications and have found your blood glucose levels increasing, it may be due to thiazide diuretics, beta blockers, or calcium channel blockers. Medications used for other purposes

TAKING MEDICATION—
IS IT NECESSARY?

can also raise blood glucose. Some medications can make the oral diabetes medications more potent, lowering blood glucose.

Depending on their mechanism for action, other diabetes medications may cause nausea, flatulence, bloating, or diarrhea. Some of these side effects will occur when you first take the medications and may decrease or disappear over time. If you are having side effects from your medications, be sure to tell your health care provider. Your diabetes team can work with you to minimize the discomfort while maximizing the drug effects.

It's best to find out about possible side effects before you take your first dose. For some medications, your doctor will start on a small dose and gradually increase the dose. This is called titration, and should help ease some of the side effects. It is important to allow enough time for it to have its full therapeutic effect. For example, metformin or acarbose may be titrated over weeks to minimize adverse events.

Your body may need time to adjust to a new medication. Ask how long you should wait before calling to report symptoms. If the side effect is unbearable, call your health care provider. There are often other options available, so speak up, but never stop taking a drug without speaking with your diabetes care team first.

As you are prescribed new medications, be sure to ask about side effects, adverse events, and when you should report the effects of a new medication to the office. When you start a new medication and find your blood glucose is higher or lower, check to be sure it is not due to your new medication.

WEEK 3	Appointments with Your Diabetes Team

Health care visits can be stressful and confusing for many people. Before your next appointment, there are a few things you can do to prepare, allowing you to get the most from your visit. Bring to your appointment a copy of the medication record you worked on in Week 1.

WHAT TO TAKE TO YOUR APPOINTMENT

Medication list (prescription and nonprescription)

Brown bag of all medications

Blood glucose log

Monitoring supplies

Note pad and pencil

List of all questions

Another method to accomplish this is to place all your medications in a small brown paper bag and take it to the doctor's office with you. Remember to include any over-the-counter medications that you are taking. This method often catches a number of potential causes for less than optimal blood glucose. Some of the common mistakes include taking medications more or less frequently than prescribed or taking them at the wrong time, like at meals when they should be taken on an empty stomach. Another common mistake is taking a medication that was stopped, when a different medication should have replaced it. Even taking vitamins or herbal supplements can affect your blood glucose or interfere with the prescription medications you are taking. Take the list of questions you have, along with a notepad to write down the answers.

Another issue you may want to address at this visit is the cost of prescription medications and supplies. Out-of-pocket expenses are soaring, and people who have diabetes bear a greater burden. Even with insurance, personal health care costs are rising annually.

Along with your normal health care visits, you should schedule an annual medication review with at least one of the members of your diabetes care team. This is an excellent opportunity for you to speak up

TAKING MEDICATION—
IS IT NECESSARY?

about any problems you are having. You need to be honest about your problems because there are solutions to most of your difficulties. Allow your health care team to make suggestions to help you improve your control. Remember that you will need to take some time to prepare for your appointment. Write down your concerns and discuss the questions you have regarding your medications and diabetes health plan. Your goal may be to simplify your routine, reduce costs when possible, or understand what you are taking and why.

Diabetes is all about self-care. Medications are critical to your care. You play the greatest role in managing your diabetes medications. The purpose of this annual review is to ask questions about your medications. Possible questions to ask yourself before the appointment are:

- Is the medication schedule too complicated or too time consuming for you?

- Are you having difficulties swallowing certain pills, or do they upset your stomach?

- Do you know the names of your medications and understand how they all work?

- If you take a lot of pills during the day, is it common to mix them up? When should I take my many medications?

- Is the cost of medication a problem for you? If so, ask the doctor if there is a generic version of the medication you could take or if the medication is available in a combination pill.

Your health care team will have the answers to your questions and solutions to any problems you may experience. Don't be afraid to ask!

Have you ever said, "Did I take my pills this morning?" Remembering to take your medications can be a problem. Everyone will miss a dose here or there, but many people need help to jog their memory on a regular basis. If your memory needs a little help, there are numerous tricks, devices, and gadgets available.

5 STEPS TO REMEMBERING TO TAKE YOUR MEDICATION

1. Organize your medications in one spot.
2. Link your dose to a daily event (i.e., brushing your teeth, eating breakfast, etc.).
3. Keep a log of when you took your medication.
4. Set a daily timer to go off when it's time for a dose (watch, clock, cell phone).
5. Use a weekly or monthly pill box to organize and visually tell you if you took a dosage.

Here are several suggestions to help you remember to take your medication. Begin by organizing your medications in one spot. You are more likely to remember to take your medications if they are all together and in a place you are likely to be at the time your dose is due. If you link taking your medication with an activity or event, you are more likely to remember and not miss a dose. An example would be taking your medication while brushing your teeth in the morning or evening. By doing this, you will form a mental habit that makes it easier to remember.

Writing down medications will often help, as well. Check the medication off the chart every time you take a dose. Use a calendar to keep track of medications, marking the calendar when you take each medication. If remembering to take medications on time is a problem, set a timer on your watch, clock, computer, or cell phone to

TAKING MEDICATION—
IS IT NECESSARY?

remind you when a dose is due. This works particularly well if some doses are scheduled at odd times of the day. Using a weekly (seven day) pill box with days of the week is a great method because you can see the pills laid out for each day, making it easy to see if you forgot to take a medication. Also available are monthly pill boxes to organize a 30-day supply of your medications. Pharmacies sometimes will provide a service where your pills come in prepackaged doses by time of day or day of the week.

It isn't easy in our busy and sometimes chaotic lives, but taking your medications correctly is worth the effort by maximizing your glucose control. Maintaining a consistent schedule of eating, exercise, and medications helps you to better identify patterns, and adjust your treatments for optimal health. If you continue to have problems remembering to take your medications, look to simplify your medication therapy. Discuss with your health care provider ways to decrease the many medications you are taking. Some medications combine two different drugs into one pill. There are a variety of combination pills currently available.

For your medications to maintain their potency, it is important to store them properly. The majority of medications should be stored in a cool, dry environment. Many people store their medications in the bathroom, where conditions are often hot and steamy, causing the medication to lose potency and not work as effectively. To determine how to store medication, read the labels on medication containers and pharmacy printouts when picking up your prescriptions. Manufacturers of insulin, exenatide, and pramlintide recommend storing these in a refrigerator prior to use. You may keep these medications safely at room temperature for about a month. Once opened, follow manufacturers instructions for storage. The medication printout contains valuable information about the medication, including how to store each medication to maintain its efficacy.

Syringes, needles, and lancets for blood glucose monitoring are considered medical equipment. If you are using medical equipment, you will need to know how to safely dispose of the syringes, needles, and lancets. States and counties have different regulations for disposal of medical equipment. Sometimes guidelines can be found on your pharmacy printout. If not, you can contact the county board of health for information, or ask you pharmacist or any member of your health care team. In general, use a red sharps disposal container for disposal of needles and syringes. These containers can be found at your local pharmacy.

SIMPLE MEDICATION MANAGEMENT TIPS

- Save the pharmacy printouts and place them with your medical records. You may want to consider keeping a notebook or folder that includes this information.

- Shop for a pharmacy that has hours when you want to shop. Use a store where a pharmacist is available to answer questions, and will take an interest in your medical needs. Consult with your pharmacist for an annual medication review.

- Consult your health care provider before switching to a different type or brand of insulin.

The cost of health care is rising. The cost of medication for type 2 diabetes is often a barrier for people taking their medications as prescribed. Don't let the cost become a barrier for you taking your medications. It is important to discuss any spending limits you may have with your doctor before he prescribes a specific medication. Don't discontinue a medication or change a prescribed medication in an effort to reduce costs without first discussing it with your health care team. There are alternatives to reducing costs rather than discontinuing the medications critical to your health.

Begin by looking carefully at your health insurance plan and the cost of office visits, lab tests, vaccines, and co-payments. Look at the medications you are taking and compare them to what is covered in your plan. As you review your plan, note that preferred medications are usually less expensive than others. What are the co-payments? With so many insurance plans available, health care providers don't know what is covered under every plan when they are prescribing medications. Bring a list of covered medications with you to the office and review them with your physician. With the list in hand, it is easier to ask about alternatives that would cost less.

Your pharmacist can also make recommendations of lower cost drugs offered by your health plan. Many employers who offer sponsored insurance have an open season, a time when you are allowed to move in and out of insurance plans. If you are choosing a new plan, it is a good idea to list out and compare the services and medications you need and use on an annual basis.

Shopping around for the best prices for medications and supplies can save you a great deal. The larger stores generally have lower prices. Some health plans offer a mail-order option for medications and supplies, allowing a 90-day supply versus a 30-day supply with the same co-pay, reducing the cost over time. When looking for lower prices on your medications, be careful about online pharmacies. There is a risk of counterfeit drugs, which can be dangerous, so look for a Verified Internet Pharmacy Practice Site seal of approval.

Financial assistance for medications may be available from some pharmaceutical companies. They offer free medication to people who qualify for a processing fee. Ask your health care provider or pharmacist about these programs.

Another strategy to spend less could be the use of combination oral agents. There are varieties available containing two pills in one. Always ask if there is a generic equivalent when a new medication is prescribed. The generic medications are lower in price, cutting some of your out-of-pocket costs. Use the time during your medication review to talk with your doctor about cutting out any unnecessary or less effective medications.

Everyone will miss a dose of medication once in a while. Given the complexity of diabetes, that can be expected. It is not uncommon when you have diabetes to feel that you cannot possibly do something recommended by your diabetes health care team. Many people can't remember to take a medication at the correct time. It may be that you don't have regular work or sleep hours because of the type of work you do. Maybe you don't take or forget to take medications because you are embarrassed to take them in a public place. For many women with school-aged children, 3 p.m. begins a never-ending cycle of homework, after-school activities, dinner, and bath and bed time. It is easy to get lost in the many demands placed on top of your diabetes. Another barrier could be visual; you can't read the label or see the syringe. Cost of the medication can be another large barrier, causing you to cut pills in half or take a dose every other day instead of daily.

Your diabetes care team is under the assumption that you are taking your medication as prescribed. If you are not reaching blood glucose, lipid, or blood pressure levels within the targeted range, they will assume the medication is not working effectively and may increase doses or change timing to help you reach your goal. This begins a cycle of adjustments that will not improve the way you feel or help you reach the targeted levels to prevent or delay complications.

Take a few moments and look honestly at the cause of missed doses. Write your reasons in your log book and share these with your health care providers at your next visit. If you have a vision or dexterity problem and can't manage without the assistance of someone else, there are a number of devices—magnifiers, larger print for labeling medications, syringe-filling devices—that can help you. If your schedule is the issue, perhaps a change in medication or its timing can be prescribed. If you have financial concerns because of the cost of your diabetes medication or all your medications combined, there is assistance for medication programs or generic brands available that can help decrease the cost.

Explain to your diabetes care team what barriers are keeping you from taking your medications as prescribed. There are many solutions available for any given problem that arises. Remember technology, techniques (skills), and medications are continuously being improved.

Traveling with diabetes takes a little extra thought and planning. You may feel overwhelmed by what could happen when traveling, but most obstacles can be planned for and resolved. Diabetes should never be a reason for you not to travel.

TRAVELING TIPS

Here are some tips that will ensure a stress-free trip whether it is for pleasure or work related.

- Be sure to wear a medical ID bracelet or necklace identifying that you have diabetes in case of an emergency.
- Obtain copies of all your prescriptions, packing them in your carry-on in case you need a refill while away from home.
- The name and phone number of your pharmacy should also be included somewhere that you have access to at all times.
- Carry your medications in your carry-on bag to prevent loss in your checked luggage or separation in the case of a mislaid bag.
- Be sure to take the prescription label for your diabetes supplies (for example, the pharmacy label is found on the box of injectible medications).
- It is a good idea to ask for a letter from your doctor that includes your name, your diagnosis of diabetes, and a list of all your medications and supplies (blood glucose monitoring supplies such as strips, lancets, alcohol, etc). Have your physician sign and date the letter. If you use insulin or have an insulin pump, be sure to include in the letter the name of your pump, infusion sets, needles, syringes, vials of insulin, and pens or other devices.

Occasionally you may miss a meal while traveling due to missed connections or arrive at a hotel too late for room service. Be prepared for all circumstances. You should pack snacks to supplement or replace a meal that is missed. Crackers and cheese or peanut butter, granola bars, and fruit cups are easy to pack and travel well. Depending on the length of your trip and availability to restock your supplies while traveling, try to pack up two meals per day while traveling.

Traveling by air? Besides the stress of tickets, connecting flights, hotel reservations, and auto rentals, you will have to deal with the Transportation Security Administration (TSA), a division of the U.S. Department of Homeland Security. For some people with diabetes, this stops them from traveling by air. Don't let it stop you from any adventure you wish to undertake.

It is important to keep your medical items in your carry-on luggage. Separate out supplies and equipment related to your diabetes and tell the TSA agent at the security gate about your needs. Learning the guidelines for air travel before you go can help relieve any apprehensions you may have about traveling.

TSA-PERMITTED LIQUIDS FOR PERSONS WITH MEDICAL CONDITIONS

TSA permits prescription liquid medications and other liquids needed by people with medical conditions that include:

- All prescription and over-the-counter medications (liquids, gels, and aerosols) for medical purposes.
- Liquids including water, juice, or liquid nutrition or gels for a medical condition.
- Gels or frozen liquids needed to cool medical-related items for medical conditions.

If the liquid medications are in volumes larger than 3 ounces, they may not be placed in a quart size bag, and they must be declared to the TSA officer. A declaration can be made verbally, in writing, or by a person's traveling companion.

Declared liquids must be kept separate from all other property and submitted for x-ray screening.

www.tsa.gov/travelers/airtravel/specialneeds/index.shtm. Accessed October 20, 2007

| CHAPTER 6 | Tackling the Problem Head On |

The day-to-day management of your diabetes is up to you. There are a number of self-care activities that everyone with diabetes must understand to avoid the daily problems that can occur when living with diabetes. To avoid problems, you will need to recognize and then respond to a number of situations, including hyperglycemia, hypoglycemia, and sick day management. Responding effectively to problems as they present themselves will take both knowledge and skills. Therefore, to tackle the possible day-to-day problems of living with diabetes, you must first learn as much as you can about diabetes.

In people without diabetes, the body has a self-regulating glucose control system. It works to maintain blood glucose within normal levels of 65–99 mg/dL, preventing glucose from rising too high or dropping too low. Normally, the foods you eat break down into glucose and enter your bloodstream. As the levels of glucose increase, a signal is sent for the pancreas to make and secrete the hormone insulin. Insulin enters the bloodstream, allowing glucose to enter the body cells (muscle, liver, and fat tissues). As glucose enters the cells, it is used for energy and the amount stored in the blood stream decreases. The drop in glucose in the bloodstream signals the pancreas to stop secreting insulin. Secretion of the right amount of insulin maintains blood glucose within normal ranges. Glucose is then used as energy or stored for energy use at a later time in the absence of glucose or insulin. This process is an automatic response, like breathing; we do not need to think about it.

As type 2 diabetes develops, the defects are twofold: The body either produces too little insulin, or the body and muscle cells ignore or resist the action of insulin. The skeletal muscle, liver, and adipose (fat) tissues are the primary sites of the insulin resistance. Insulin resistance occurs when the body fails to use available insulin properly.

Maintaining normal blood glucose control with type 2 diabetes will require matching the timing of medications to mimic the insulin secretion from the pancreas. Medications are prescribed with a preset dose and action, which means meal planning and activity need to remain consistent to ensure a somewhat predictable blood glucose elevation to maintain normal blood glucose levels. Type 2 diabetes is a progressive disease with insulin production decreasing over the first 5–10 years. One goal of treatment is to restore and optimize glycemic control. For all the wonderful advancements that have been made in the treatment of type 2 diabetes in the past 10 years, current medications and devices have limited ability to duplicate normal insulin production. While treatments are greatly improved, they are not perfect. Therefore, you can expect to tackle some of the more common problems like hyperglycemia and hypoglycemia.

Attending a diabetes self-management training program will provide you with the tools for the prevention and treatment of the occasional problem. With knowledge and experience over time, you will find that you are both comfortable and confident to handle any problem. Work with your diabetes educator on your diabetes care team several times a year to evaluate target goals, make adjustments in your management plan, and review your self-management skills. Your educator will make sure that you feel comfortable to handle daily decisions that help you maintain blood glucose within range. Managing fluctuations in blood glucose levels will take ongoing decisions about your food and activity choices and medication adjustments. This approach to diabetes management includes identifying the problem, working toward your set target goals, and developing a diabetes care plan. Your care plan is a tool for problem-solving based on your health care provider's recommendations but tailored to your individual lifestyle. The diabetes care plan will become more refined as it evolves over time. Daily management of diabetes is up to you, but you are not alone. You have the support of your diabetes care team.

Although it is not always possible, prevention is the best method to avoid serious problems with your diabetes. Maintaining blood glucose control is one aspect of preventive care. Following your meal plan, remaining physically active, and taking your medications correctly are key to avoiding problems in the first place. However, even with your best efforts, you will experience fluctuations such as hyperglycemia and hypoglycemia.

When you look at the common diabetes problems in this chapter, realize they are short term in nature, typically appearing in hours or days. These problems develop rapidly and respond to treatment just as quickly. These problems, when handled, are preventable and if you cannot prevent them from occurring they are quickly treatable. These complications of diabetes can temporarily affect your ability to function normally. For example, you may have trouble focusing or thinking clearly. When you are in control of your diabetes, the short-term problems are avoidable. In these eight weeks, you will be presented with strategies to prevent and treat these common problems.

Hyperglycemia is a factor in the development of long-term complications. Recommended fasting capillary blood glucose levels are 70–130 mg/dL. Ask your health care provider for your individual target numbers for blood glucose if you do not already know your target range. Recognizing and responding to the symptoms of hyperglycemia promptly will enable you to reduce or avoid complications. Below are some of the common symptoms of high blood glucose. It is important that you are aware of the symptoms and recognize those you commonly experience.

SYMPTOMS OF AND TREATMENTS FOR HYPERGLYCEMIA

If you have these symptoms, hyperglycemia, you are no doubt outside your suggested target ranges and you need to take action. What should you do?

Symptoms:

- Excessive thirst or hunger
- Frequent urination, especially at night
- A tired or sleepy feeling
- Lack of energy
- Blurred vision
- Frequent infections
- Slow healing of cuts or sores
- Dry or itchy skin

Treatments:

- Check your blood glucose and record in your monitor log
- Test your blood glucose more frequently and record
- Take your correct dose of medication at the right time
- Follow your meal plan

The cause of high blood glucose can involve one or several factors. These are the common reasons for high blood glucose:

- Forgot to take your medications

- Not taking enough diabetes medication

TACKLING THE PROBLEM
HEAD ON

- Eating too much or more calories than you use for energy

- Not exercising enough or regularly

- Another medical condition, such as infection

In the absence of an infection, getting back to the basics (a balance of medications, meal planning, and activity) will correct high blood glucose by lowering it back within your target range. If blood glucose continues to climb with physical symptoms to levels above 240 mg/dL, call your health care provider. Be sure to check your blood glucose monitoring system to ensure your meter is working correctly, so that you are getting accurate readings. Check to see if your monitoring system needs to be cleaned some need periodic maintenance. Check the accuracy of your meter with control solutions. When you opened new strips, did you enter the code? Newer meters no longer require this step. Check to see if the strips have expired. Look at your medications to see if they have changed in color or appearance, indicating they have lost potency or the medication has expired. In your log book, list your symptoms, what you have eaten, and the medications you have taken, including the name and dose.

Actions that lower blood glucose levels in the absence of illness or infection include an increase or change in the type of medication you are taking, eating less, and/or exercising more.

Prolonged hyperglycemia

Prolonged hyperglycemia (high blood glucose) can lead to diabetic ketoacidosis (DKA) or hyperosmolar hyperglycemic nonketotic syndrome (HHNS). HHNS is a combination of hyperglycemia and dehydration, much like DKA. Blood glucose can reach levels over 600 mg/dL. DKA only occurs when there is a deficiency of insulin. DKA occurs more often in type 1 diabetes but it can occur in people with type 2. Those with type 2 will develop ketoacidosis only when they have severe infections or trauma that places their bodies under great physical stress. DKA is a combination of major hyperglycemia, dehydration, acidosis, and ketosis. Prompt medical attention is necessary to avoid the serious condition that may lead to a change in mental state, leading to a loss of consciousness and possible death. Symptoms of ketoacidosis include nausea, vomiting, extreme tiredness, weakness, and dehydration.

Prevention of DKA or HHNS begins with self-management training teaching you how to recognize the symptoms and take action, such as monitoring your blood glucose levels. If your blood glucose is greater than 240 mg/dL, you may want to check your urine for ketones. Ketones are chemical compounds produced when fats are used for energy instead of carbohydrates. In the absence of insulin, your body cannot use glucose in your bloodstream for energy. Ketones are a by-product of burning stored fat for energy when you are not eating carbohydrates, when sleeping, or on a low carbohydrate diet. People who have hyperglycemia and elevated blood ketones (ketosis) have ketoacidosis. Ketones become dangerous when they build to extremely high levels in the blood. If you have elevated blood glucose levels and your urine is positive for ketones, call your physician immediately. Illnesses like acute infections can trigger DKA. Influenza, other respiratory tract infections, and gastroenteritis are common causes of DKA; therefore, special care is necessary when you are experiencing an illness. Beware of the symptoms of high blood glucose levels, check blood glucose levels regularly, follow your sick day guidelines, and report results to your health care provider when you are not within your glucose target range.

Hypoglycemia is a condition of low blood glucose, and is the result of elevated amounts of insulin lowering blood glucose to low levels. Hypoglycemia is a consequence of your diabetes medications and treatments. Unfortunately, the treatments and therapies for diabetes are not perfect and sometimes blood glucose will drop too low when insulin is elevated in the bloodstream. It can occur if you take too much medication, exercise too long, or eat too little by skipping meals. Hypoglycemia can be conservatively defined as blood glucose levels of 70 mg/dL or less with symptoms, but individual people have different levels at which they will become symptomatic. The duration of diabetes does play a role at what level you will feel symptomatic. Some people with a long-time duration of diabetes may not even recognize low blood glucose if symptoms present themselves.

Low blood glucose reactions are categorized as mild or severe. A mild reaction results in symptoms like sweating, trembling, lightheadedness,

SYMPTOMS OF AND TREATMENTS FOR HYPOGLYCEMIA

Symptoms:

- Irritability
- Sweaty
- Shaky or jittery
- Rapid heartbeat
- Hunger
- Headache
- Confusion
- Double vision
- Fatigue
- Tingling sensation around the mouth
- Pale skin color

Treatments:

15 grams of glucose or carbohydrates:

- 8 oz of nonfat skim milk
- 1/2 cup or 4 oz regular soda (not sugar free)
- 1/2 cup or 4 oz fruit juice
- 3–4 glucose tablets
- 1 dose of glucose gel
- 1 Tbsp of honey or sugar

and difficulty concentrating. Symptoms can be quickly identified and treated by drinking or eating carbohydrates. A severe reaction is when people are unable to treat themselves because of confusion or unconsciousness. Because of the inability to self-treat, others must provide the treatment to raise your blood glucose levels. The majority of hypoglycemic cases are mild reactions, especially for those with type 2 diabetes.

If you develop these symptoms, act quickly. Check your blood glucose then treat with one of the suggested treatments of 15 grams of glucose or carbohydrate. Wait 15–20 minutes and recheck your blood sugars. If you are still experiencing low blood glucose, repeat the treatment and consume 15 grams of carbohydrates until your blood glucose increases 30–45 mg/dL. Everyone responds individually. If you are unsure of your symptoms or you cannot check your blood glucose level, it's better to treat your hypoglycemia than it is to wait it out.

There are several factors that will increase the risk for hypoglycemia in type 2 diabetes, including advancing age, poor nutritional status, and hepatic (liver) or renal (kidney) disease. Anyone who takes certain oral medications or insulin can have low blood glucose reactions. Some are at a greater risk because they are taking insulin or medications that produce more insulin and lower blood glucose. Being prepared is the key to preventing serious cases of hypoglycemia. You should always carry a small portion of food or another source of glucose with you in case you have a low blood glucose reaction.

Everyone will occasionally develop the common cold, flu, or stomach viruses. If you have diabetes, you will need to take some extra precaution to keep your blood glucose within your target range. Your diabetes care team will work to provide you with sick day instructions, which are guidelines for managing your illness at home.

If you have been given sick day guidelines it is a good idea to review them periodically. A good time to review them is in the early fall, prior to cold and flu season. This way, you can be sure to have the necessary items ready for whenever sickness occurs.

Here is a list of suggested items to have at home.

- Clear fluids—regular soda, ginger ale, and Sprite

- Regular Jell-O, pudding, applesauce

- Soups

- Crackers

- Icy pops (frozen popsicles in plastic)

- Anti-diarrheal medications

- Cough syrup

- Thermometer

- Pain relievers

- Cold pills

- Ketone testing strips

- Glucose monitor and testing supplies

- Log book to record testing and intake

GENERAL SICK DAY GUIDELINES

- Check your blood glucose at least every two hours while awake.
- Drink plenty of fluids. If your temperature is over 99° drink 8 ounces of fluid every hour while awake.
- Take your oral diabetes medications, except those you take only when you eat.
- Take your usual doses of insulin if prescribed. Do not skip a dose.
- Replace the amount of carbohydrates that you eat at each meal if you cannot eat as usual. Eat carbohydrate snacks or small frequent meals consisting of 15 grams of carbohydrate like:

6–8 saltine crackers

1 slice of bread

1 cup yogurt

1 cup chicken soup

1/2 cup apple juice

Keeping a copy of your sick day guidelines and these necessary items in a plastic container with a lid is a great way to be certain you have everything you need in one easy-to-find place. It is a good idea to keep some simple foods on hand to prepare when you are not feeling well. If you prepare in advance, you won't need to make an extra trip out when you are feeling your worst.

Above is an example of general guidelines for days you are not feeling well. Your health care team will provide you with specific information for sick days, including how to handle your diabetes medications.

CALL YOUR HEALTH CARE TEAM IMMEDIATELY IF:

- You are vomiting
- You have diarrhea
- Your blood glucose is over 300 mg/dL and you are positive for ketones
- You have had a fever for more than one day
- You have a fever over 101°F
- You are dehydrated with dry mouth and cracked lips
- You have been sick for more than two days
- You have been unable to eat for more than one day
- You are having chest pain or trouble breathing

BEFORE YOU CALL YOUR HEALTH CARE TEAM, HAVE THIS INFORMATION READY:

- How long have you been sick?
- What are your symptoms?
- What are your blood glucose numbers?
- What were your ketone testing results?
- What are your temperatures?
- What have you had to eat and drink over the last 24 hours?
- Do you have your pharmacist's phone number? (Check to see if the pharmacy is open if you are calling in the evening or on the weekend.)

Living and thriving with diabetes will require active self-management. Diabetes self-management training at the time of diagnosis is important to your development of knowledge and skills to handle your diabetes on a daily basis. 95% of diabetes care will be self-care. Self-management focuses on making and acting on choices on a regular basis. At the time of diagnosis, you are often overwhelmed with information. The process for effective self-management includes learning about diabetes, defining goals, and determining the benefits and risks of treatment options. It also includes those skills necessary to achieve your choices and evaluate them periodically.

A good example of a skill is organization. Say you were given sick day guidelines at the time of your diagnosis, but two years later you come down with the flu or a nasty cold and actually need to use sick day guidelines. Chances are you don't even remember where you put those written guidelines. Diabetes self-management training is continually needed to reinforce learning and skills. Both your treatment goals and your therapies will change over time and diabetes self-management training will help you make sense of those changes.

Diabetes self-management training is patient-centered, meaning it is tailored to your medical needs, your preferences, and your social environment. There are a great number of self-care tasks that a person with diabetes must master. Realistically, simply being given all the information and skills does not mean you will be able to follow your diabetes team's recommendations. Sometimes there are too many competing demands that keep you from mastering your self-care. A good example is a recommendation of walking 30 minutes a day for five days. You know that it will help you lose weight, feel better about yourself, improve your blood glucose control, decrease your cardiovascular risks, and improve your circulation, but it is hard to find the time to fit it into your schedule. Here is an example where good communication with your team is vital to your success.

TACKLING THE PROBLEM
HEAD ON

Your team can suggest other physical activities that might be more enjoyable or ways to fit the 30 minutes into your daily life. Self-management education can simplify many of those recommendations and help prioritize them based on the areas you wish to improve.

To prevent short-term problems and learn to tackle them head on, see a diabetes educator on a regular basis. You can find a diabetes educator online through the American Association of Diabetes Educators website (www.diabeteseducator.org). This site is easy to use and, in most cases, will provide a number of qualified health care professionals with complete contact information. To find an American Diabetes Association recognized education program in your area, you can call 1-800-342-2383 or use the American Diabetes Association website (www.diabetes.org/recognition/education).

Diabetes may affect many parts of your body, so keeping your blood glucose in target range will give you more energy, help you physically feel great, and let you know that you are in control of your diabetes for life. An important aspect of prevention of short-term complications is seeking regular care with your diabetes health care team. Routine care will prevent problems by identifying them early so they can be managed.

Here are some simple things you can do to manage and prevent complications:

- Have a healthy meal plan

- Take your medications as your health care provider recommends

- Monitor your blood glucose

- Treat high blood glucose

- Treat low blood glucose

- Get regular exercise

- Perform daily foot exams

Review your monitoring log/journal to see how you are doing in each of these areas. If you are having difficulties, it may be time to seek assistance from the appropriate member of your diabetes care team.

Regular appointments with your health care team will ensure your ability to prevent possible problems. At your next regular visit, review their target recommendations for your daily fasting blood glucose and two hour post-meal blood glucose target levels. Discuss what you should do when you have elevated blood glucose levels in the absence of an illness. Review your monitoring log with your team and look for patterns in the variations from day to day and week to week. Are your fasting blood glucose levels getting higher and higher since your last visit? Compare your target fasting to your actual numbers. It may indicate you need a medication change. Depending on your monitoring schedule, you may be occasionally checking two hour post-meal blood glucose levels. How do your results compare to your target numbers? When you are not within your recommended target ranges, you may need to discuss medication, meal plans, or activity changes.

Review your sick day guidelines with your team. A good time to do this is just prior to cold and flu season every year. Many times, several years will pass since you received the sick day guidelines. Your medication and treatments may have changed substantially during that time. If you have used your sick day guidelines with success or had problems in the past, be sure to let your team know. This is a prevention measure to ensure your ability to manage a sick day or a bout of flu at home. Be sure to get a flu shot every year to increase your chances of avoiding the flu.

Staying on top of potential problems before they occur will bring you great rewards. Over time, with your health care team's guidance, you will develop the skills to manage all possible day-to-day fluctuations in your blood glucose levels. Ask as many questions as you need to understand your diabetes plan. You have a team of health care professionals behind you.

As you experience an episode of hyperglycemia or hypoglycemia, take time after to record the steps you followed. In your journal, note the symptoms, your blood glucose level, and your actions. This will help you share with your care team how well you are able to handle problems at home. Your experience is important in building skills and self-confidence in managing your diabetes.

To maintain blood glucose within your target goals here are some strategies that work:

• Check your blood glucose on a regular basis.

• Review your log every two weeks looking for patterns.

• Set appropriate target goals.

• Check your medication and eating schedule. When is your medication working its hardest to lower your blood glucose?

• Match medications to your schedule with the help of your health care team.

Over time, these may be areas you will need to address.

TACKLING THE PROBLEM
HEAD ON

Having diabetes can put you at risk. As a safety precaution, it is important to wear some type of diabetes identification to alert others that you have diabetes in the event that you cannot speak for yourself. Diabetes identification comes in a large variety, giving you many choices. They usually have a medical emblem so they stand out clearly. Medical jewelry is available in bracelets, necklaces, and pendants for both men and women. The jewelry can be found in sterling silver, 10 or 14 karat gold, nylon, or leather. If you have a more active lifestyle, you may want a durable sport band identification made of nylon or leather cuffs with an identification face plate. Medical identification is readily available at a wide range of prices. These can be found in a number of diabetes magazines and journals, at your pharmacy, at department store jewelry counters, or on order forms in your health care providers' offices.

Even when wearing diabetes identification, it is important to instruct those around you on how to recognize your usual symptoms and how to respond in case of a severe low blood glucose reaction. Be sure that your family, friends, coworkers, and others know how to recognize and treat hypoglycemia. Don't be shy. They will be happy to help. It may even be helpful to have a short list of instructions ready to go in case of an emergency.

As a precaution, the best practice is always carrying a rapid-acting glucose with you in case of low blood glucose reactions. The options here are endless, and range from hard candies to glucose tabs to gels. Look in your local pharmacy at the large variety of flavors, sizes, and consistencies available.

When you have diabetes, driving is a safety concern you need to consider. For most people, driving is an important aspect to making a living, so it is important for you to maintain a good driving record. If you have diabetes and take medication to lower your blood glucose, some special precautions should be addressed. Be aware that many states require identification of diabetes on the license. States track accident causes.

As a safety precaution, no one treated with oral agents or insulin should travel without readily available snacks or quick-acting carbohydrates. Be prepared and keep snacks in the car. Check your blood glucose level prior to driving. When you are traveling long distances by car, check your blood glucose at regular intervals. Do not skip or delay meals while driving. If you start experiencing symptoms, pull the car off the road, check your blood glucose, treat, and recheck before driving. Having a cell phone available in case of emergencies is a good safety measure. An accident caused by hypoglycemia is still the responsibility of the driver. Take action quickly if you feel symptomatic while driving. When you are hypoglycemic, boats, motorcycles, three wheelers, snowmobiles, and other powered vehicles are no less dangerous than cars.

TACKLING THE PROBLEM
HEAD ON

| CHAPTER 7 | Positive Steps to Healthy Coping |

Among chronic diseases, diabetes is unique in the amount of attention a person must devote to remaining healthy. Self-care activities are necessary for the short- and long-term benefits to your good health and quality of life. Self-care activities for diabetes include a number of lifestyle changes, such as meal planning, exercise or activity, and taking medications; all are essential to maintaining blood glucose in a healthy target range.

The first step to developing healthy coping skills is to recognize that self-care behaviors may feel difficult or challenging at times. As a person with diabetes, you may experience a wide range of feelings about managing your diabetes. It is normal to feel angry, frightened, or overwhelmed, even to the point of denying that you have diabetes. These feelings are normal when you consider the scope of diabetes. This chronic disease will be with you for the rest of your life and requires around-the-clock responsibility. Expressing your feelings to your family, friends, and your diabetes care team is an essential step to healthy coping with diabetes. Although you need to actively participate in decision making, goal setting, and daily management, you are not without support. You are not expected to cope alone. You have a care team to help you manage all aspects of living with diabetes. This level of involvement over time can be difficult for you as a person with diabetes, regardless of how motivated you are to live a long, healthy, and independent life.

We live in a complex world. Everyone experiences problems even if they do not have diabetes. Our lives are full of things that can cause stress, and each person reacts differently to the many stressors we encounter daily, including family, children, work, school, looming deadlines, finances, or changes in physical and mental health. Stress can occur from major life events, like mourning the loss of someone close to you, divorce, changing jobs, moving, getting married, the birth of your child, or the chronic care of diabetes.

Any event can cause stress, even a happy event. These stressors can take their toll over time. Everyone has an experience they could share about stressful times in their life. Studies have shown that exposure to long-term stress can shorten your life if not managed correctly. Stress is the body's response to keep you alive. When you are faced with a perceived danger, the body will release the stress hormones epinephrine (adrenaline) and cortisol. These hormones make you feel more alert and ready to react and are often referred to as flight or fight hormones. The release of epinephrine and cortisol will increase your heart rate and raise your blood pressure. The liver will release glycogen, which converts into glucose, giving your muscles rapid energy. If you are in danger, you can run to escape, but if you are stressing over traffic, waiting for an appointment, or an argument you have had with a friend, you are left with extra blood glucose. For those who don't have diabetes, the body will release insulin and lower the blood glucose automatically; however, those with diabetes may find themselves experiencing symptoms of hyperglycemia.

SYMPTOMS OF STRESS

Stress can affect everything from your blood glucose control to your ability to getting a sound night's sleep. Stress can sneak up on you. Subtle symptoms of stress include:

- frustration
- irritability
- forgetfulness
- anxiety
- insomnia

If you dealing with a constant level of low-grade stress, you may not even be aware you are dealing with stress until obvious physical symptoms present themselves. Constant stress can put your health at risk by raising your blood pressure and cholesterol, compromising your immune system, and causing gastrointestinal problems. Healthy diabetes coping skills are behaviors that can eliminate or modify the stressors common to you and your diabetes. The key is learning your subtle body changes to the things that cause stress and learning new ways to respond to the stress. Several studies have demonstrated that adding stress-reduction techniques to your self-management plan will improve your blood glucose control.

The emotional effects of diabetes are as overwhelming as the physical ones. Feeling sad and alone are not uncommon for anyone. If you feel this way for longer than two weeks, it's not stress, but could be depression. Depression has an even larger negative effect on people with diabetes. In fact, one in every four people with diabetes suffer with depression severe enough to require treatment.

Depression can make it difficult to manage self-care activities, and adversely affects a number of relevant self-care behaviors, including eating behaviors, physical activity levels, use of tobacco, and taking medications as prescribed. Even mild depression is associated with loss of blood glucose control, and increased risk of microvascular (eye and kidney) and macrovascular (cardiovasular disease) complications, because of the adverse effect on self-care activities and health behaviors.

With medications and counseling interventions, depression can be treated successfully. Unfortunately, depression remains unrecognized and untreated in a majority of cases. Depression is under-diagnosed in people with diabetes because the symptoms are often attributed to self-care issues, and symptoms of depression and diabetes overlap, causing confusion. These factors emphasize the importance of clear, honest communication with your health care provider and care team.

Living with diabetes can evoke strong feelings. You may feel uncertain, frustrated, resentful, or angry at times. Many feel they have no control of their lives. Look for ways to fit diabetes into your lifestyle. Explore ways that you can use every day: Talk with a supportive friend, meditate or pray, or seek the support of others—whether it is friends, family, or a member of your health care team.

Learn as much as you can about diabetes through asking questions. Knowledge is power. Learning about diabetes is a life long process, so don't expect to do it all at once. Know what works for you and what you are able and willing to do to manage your diabetes. You have made thousands of decisions about your diet, activity levels, and medications. This experience and knowledge will help you make lifestyle changes today and tomorrow.

Motivation and resilience are internal qualities found in everyone. Motivation is a process of finding an incentive that moves us to action. Think about things that have motivated you and continue to motivate you. Resiliency is your ability to recover quickly from illness, change, or misfortune. We have all met or heard of people who have overcome insurmountable odds. Can you learn from them and others to find your personal strengths? Have you handled health or other commitments well? What has inspired you in the past? Discover what makes you strong and keeps you motivated. This exercise will take some thought. Find out what keeps you motivated and use it to achieve the long-term results you want.

Continuous perfect diabetes self-care is impossible, so don't set yourself up for failure if you are having trouble with a certain part of your care. Negative self-talk can be very destructive to your wellbeing. Instead, congratulate or reward yourself for your efforts. Focus on what you are doing well.

Empowerment is having the knowledge and skills you need to succeed with your diabetes self-management. The cornerstone of the empowerment approach of diabetes management is recognizing that people with diabetes are responsible for managing their illness through choices, control, and consequences.

Everyone who lives with diabetes should have a diabetes management plan. This is a written road map or plan for your diabetes care, which clearly lays out your goals for self-care. Nothing assures self-care management success more than realistic goals, a plan of action, and achievement of your goals. This will empower you to better manage your daily choices and the consequences of those choices.

Begin by asking these questions about your diabetes control:

- What is the problem?

- How do I feel about the problem?

- What do I want to do?

- How will I do it?

- How did it work?

After thinking about what you want to do and deciding on an area of concern, it is time to set realistic goals to obtain the outcome you want for your diabetes control. A well thought through plan will get you the results you desire. One method for goal setting is SMART. SMART stands for Specific, Measurable, Achievable, Realistic, and Timing. An essential element in diabetes self-management is diabetes education. Part of the education process is goal setting. Through education you will gain the knowledge and skills necessary to problem solve, ask the important questions, and stay on top of an ever-changing therapy.

USING **SMART** TO DEVELOP YOUR GOALS

Here is how it works. We will use exercise as a goal because exercise is good for everything—it decreases blood glucose levels, decreases fat around your mid-section, improves blood flow, lowers your risk for heart attacks and stroke, and makes you feel better. Exercise is a simple and an inexpensive lifestyle behavior.

S pecific goals help break down a lofty goal and will focus your efforts. The common error in setting goals is they are too general. A common goal for many is, "I will exercise more." A better goal with the same intent would be, "I will walk 30 minutes a day."

M easurable goals will tell you when you have met the goal. "I will walk 30 minutes a day at least five days a week for the next eight weeks." At the end of eight weeks you will know if you have been successful.

A chievable goals are possible. If you are having foot surgery next week you may not achieve the goal of walking "30 minutes a day at least five days a week." It is not achievable if you have your foot in a cast.

R ealistic goals for you mean you are willing to work toward the goal and have the time and resources to make it happen. Goals are your own. There are many areas of diabetes care, so choose one that is important to you.

T iming your goal is necessary to succeed. A well thought out goal has a deadline or due date. In this case, eight weeks is the time-frame you're shooting for.

Try the SMART method to develop your own personal goal to improve your health. Write it on a sheet of paper. Is your goal specific? Can you measure the goal? Is it a realistic goal? What is your deadline? You may have several rewrites before you meet all the criteria. If you are committed to the goal, post the goal in a prominent place as a reminder. Also, be sure to share it with your diabetes team at your next visit.

Diabetes can cause stress because it requires a level of awareness, skill, and problem solving unlike most other medical conditions. One step to healthy coping with diabetes is accepting that stress will always be present. Although you may understand that changing certain lifestyle factors will greatly improve your health, replacing old habits and adopting new lifestyles is never easy. Some changes you will manage without difficulty and others will take time. The amount of time and attention required to deal with a chronic illness like diabetes is likely to cause stress at times. Realize that in today's world, stress is a factor for everyone.

You cannot rid yourself of stress, but you can learn to manage it. Stress is the physical and emotional reaction to situations that are perceived as a threat to well-being and is seen as unmanageable and beyond your control. A stressor is a condition or situation that causes the stress, and can be acute or chronic in nature. Stress can impair your ability for the self-care activities that are necessary for control of your diabetes. Long-term stress will takes its toll.

There are two types of stress. First is the positive type that makes us feel energetic and more productive. You may have a lot to do, but

SYMPTOMS OF STRESS

Physical symptoms:

- Headaches
- Muscle tension
- Back pain
- Racing heart beat
- Shortness of breath
- Chest pain
- Indigestion
- Constipation

Emotional symptoms:

- Irritability
- Anxiety
- Nervousness
- Frustration
- Difficulty thinking clearly
- Inability to make decisions
- Sleep disturbances

you feel in control and exhilarated by the experience. The second type is the complete opposite and wears you out and depletes you of energy. You may feel pressured from a number of directions. Stress may be a reflection of a variety of sources, including family, finances, work, and mental or physical problems. Your body will not distinguish between mental or physical stress. Regardless of the cause, the body's reaction will be to increase glucose to give us the energy to mobilize ourselves. The most common causes of stress in relation to diabetes are:

- Frustration at not reaching targeted goals

- Onset of long-term complications

- Expense of diabetes self-care

- Unclear goals or directions for care

- Poor interactions and relationships with health care providers

- Inadequate social support

Knowing yourself is the key to healthy coping. Think about what types of things create or trigger your own stress. There will be a number of potential causes. Diabetes treatment itself may contribute to stress. Write down the things that upset you daily. In a journal, identify the cause of your

CHECKLIST FOR STRESS

The first step to alleviating stress in your life is to recognize what factors are causing you stress. Below is a checklist of possibilities that are known to be great causes of stress. Identify which of these are stressors in your life.

- ☐ Newly diagnosed with diabetes
- ☐ Change in health status
- ☐ Change in job or work environment
- ☐ Change in family
- ☐ Learning a new skill
- ☐ Developing a complication associated with diabetes
- ☐ Traffic
- ☐ Noise
- ☐ Divorce
- ☐ Elderly parents
- ☐ Children
- ☐ Holidays
- ☐ Car trouble
- ☐ Retirement
- ☐ Grief
- ☐ Loss of…
- ☐ Separation
- ☐ Travel
- ☐ Moving

stress and how you react or you feel about the stressor. Rank those things that cause you a great deal of discomfort versus those that cause little stress.

Identifying the stressors that most directly impact you is a good start in helping you overcome the negative effects of stress. How stress affects you is unique to you, so you need to explore your individual reactions to stressful situations. Signs of physical stress include pain, cold hands, diarrhea, indigestion, racing heart, or shortness of breath. Signs of psychological stress include anxiety, forgetfulness, insomnia, and irritability.

Understand everyone is subject to stress. Stress can be managed, but first you need to recognize the cause and your physical and mental symptoms, and then apply one of a number of stress-management techniques that can reduce or prevent stress. Stress needs to be managed throughout your lifetime because of negative long-term effects on your body and emotional well-being.

Identifying and understanding the causes of your stress and how it makes you feel will help you to begin preventing stress. Learning to relax using relaxation techniques, biofeedback, meditation, or a stress-management program can prevent stress. Progressive relaxation is an effective technique that has been used to treat the symptoms of stress. It is easy to learn and doesn't require equipment or travel. It focuses on tensing and relaxing all major muscle groups in the body.

You probably have used a number of methods over your lifetime to deal with stress in your life, including a number of unhealthy choices. Think of ways you have handled stressful situations in the past and write these in your journal. Identify methods that seem to reduce your stress levels. Some of these will be positive and healthy ways to cope, while others will be negative. Negative methods of coping may relieve stress but are not healthy in the long run. Negative methods of coping include excessive alcohol consumption, excessive eating, excessive sleeping, drug use, smoking, etc. When under stress, negative thoughts make you feel helpless and less able to manage your self care. Those thoughts can become actions. If you are feeling angry, frightened, or guilty, it may infer with your diabetes management.

Your health care team will work with you to suggest the best approach for you. Counseling may help you learn to change the way you react to stress. Try to replace the negative with positive approaches. Don't think in terms of what you can't do; instead, focus on what you can do. Using the list on the next page, check the healthy methods of coping you have used. Make a list of healthy ways you may deal with stress in the future. Completing this exercise will increase your awareness of stress in your life and its causes and consequences. It will help you realize that you have been successfully managing stress.

HEALTHY WAYS TO REDUCE STRESS

- [ ] Change the way you react in some situations; it will reduce the way you feel in new or difficult situations
- [ ] Learn to relax
- [ ] Deep breathing
- [ ] Exercise to reduce the tension in your muscles
- [ ] Think positive thoughts
- [ ] Talk about it
- [ ] Put it on paper and keep a journal
- [ ] Listen to soothing music
- [ ] Soak in a tub
- [ ] Stress avoidance – learn to say no
- [ ] Laugh – rent and watch a funny movie
- [ ] Look to nature
- [ ] Eat wisely
- [ ] Get enough sleep
- [ ] Play every day
- [ ] Reading, Sudoku, or a craft project
- [ ] New positive actions (exercise)
- [ ] Increasing frequency of positive actions (exercise or self-blood glucose monitoring)
- [ ] Ceasing destructive actions (smoking)
- [ ] Maintaining positive health behaviors

At your next diabetes appointment, use your journal to talk to your health care provider or a member of the team about self-care activities or other things that seem difficult and cause you stress. For people with diabetes, there are potential stressors that commonly occur, including the diagnosis of diabetes, having to begin insulin, complications or the anticipation of complications, the risk of hypoglycemia, and taking on too many self-care behaviors at one time. When your stressors are related to self-care behaviors, be sure to share what is working or not working.

Health care professionals on your team are there to support you and can provide you with information about diabetes, teach you skills, help you set goals, and provide ongoing support. Don't be afraid that your diabetes care team will be upset or mad at you. They are not there to judge. Their goal is to help you gain control over your diabetes. They can usually suggest more than one solution to any problem you may experience with your diabetes management. Because there are many solutions, you should not feel you have failed if you are struggling. If you have tried one and it didn't work, your team will be able to suggest another strategy. Rarely is there only one way to deal with a diabetes-related concern. People have different lifestyles; therefore, they need different solutions. Over time, you may need to change your diabetes management plan. It is never easy, but most tasks or skills can be simplified and can enable you to master one aspect and then add on to each accomplishment until it becomes a habit.

To be successful at self-management of your diabetes, you will need to focus on positive thoughts and positive behavior changes. It is well understood that positive self-care behaviors, such as increasing your activity level, taking your medications as prescribed, frequent self-blood glucose monitoring, and stopping smoking, will improve your blood glucose control and ultimately your quality of life.

POSITIVE STEPS TO
HEALTHY COPING

Living with diabetes isn't easy. There will be times when you are angry and resentful about your diabetes. This is normal, but the kind of distress that changes the way you eat, sleep, or work may be depression. Depression is common in diabetes. People with diabetes are twice as likely to experience clinical depression as the general population according to several studies. In the general population, women are more likely than men to suffer depression. This remains true for those with diabetes. Depression causes some people to act in ways that interfere with glucose control, like forgetting to take their medications, smoking, making unhealthy food choices, or becoming less active.

At the cellular level, the body's response to depression is to become more insulin resistant. Insulin resistance is when the body's cells resist the action of insulin. It is insulin that allows glucose to leave the bloodstream to enter the body cells. Insulin resistance causes glucose to build up in the blood, causing hyperglycemia and loss of glucose control.

There is a strong link between diabetes and depression, so be sure you are aware of the symptoms before it impairs your blood glucose control. If you have the symptoms of depression, call your health care team and and talk with them about your symptoms. Feeling worthless, sad, sleeping more than usual, and a lack of interest in family and friends can all be symptoms. If you are depressed, there are safe and effective treatments for depression, including counseling and/or medication. Discuss all available options. Antidepressant medications are some of the most commonly prescribed drugs in the country. Antidepressants can take up to six weeks for you to notice a difference in the way you feel.

Attention to negative emotions along with the signs and symptoms of depression are positive first steps to coping. Research suggests about 25% to 50% of people with diabetes are depressed. If you identify these signs and symptoms, you need to seek help. Remember you do not need to manage depression alone.

DEPRESSION CHECKLIST

Have you experienced…?

☐ **Loss of pleasure.** You no longer take interest in doing things you used to enjoy.

☐ **Change in sleep patterns.** You have trouble falling asleep, you wake often during the night, or you want to sleep more than usual, including during the day.

☐ **Early to rise.** You wake up earlier than usual and cannot get back to sleep.

☐ **Change in appetite.** You eat more or less than you used to, resulting in a quick weight gain or weight loss.

☐ **Trouble concentrating.** You can't watch a TV program or read an article because other thoughts or feelings get in the way.

☐ **Loss of energy.** You feel tired all the time.

☐ **Nervousness.** You always feel so anxious you can't sit still.

☐ **Guilt.** You feel you "never do anything right" and worry that you are a burden to others.

☐ **Morning sadness.** You feel worse in the morning than you do the rest of the day.

☐ **Suicidal thoughts.** You feel you want to die or are thinking about ways to hurt yourself.

If you have three or more of these symptoms, or if you have just one or two but have been feeling bad for two weeks or more, **it's time to get help**.

www.diabetes.org/type2/depression.jsp. Accessed February 12, 2008.

Your diabetes care team includes health care professionals, friends, and family, who are there ready to focus on improving your health. Use your team to improve your understanding of diabetes. Your team is there to guide and support you. Do not hesitate; tell them honestly if you are struggling with a recommended goal for therapy or taking your medication. Take your journal to your appointments to share how things have gone since your last visit.

Your team is not going to judge. It is difficult to change your lifestyle, especially if you need to lose weight and exercise. Everyone struggles with lifestyle changes even when they have had diabetes for a long time. Your team wants to see you succeed and they are there to help. The doctor who made your diagnosis of diabetes was mostly likely your primary care physician. In most medical communities, the primary care physician is the cornerstone for managing your diabetes. In your journal, make a list of health care professionals and others who are on your diabetes health care team.

COMMON HEALTHY COPING PROBLEMS TO EXPLORE WITH TEAM

- Inaccurate understanding about diabetes
- Difficulties with food and eating habits
- Competing priorities in your life
- Stress
- Family problems
- Depression
- Feelings about diabetes

Some problems may be uncomfortable to discuss. You may have some concerns and feel ashamed or embarrassed so you wish to seek other professionals. Perhaps you are sleeping poorly or are very anxious. You may decide to see a mental health professional. A mental health professional can help you cope with stress, explore a bout with depression, or decrease or prevent stress that is related to your diabetes treatment and care. How can you find one if there is not one on your team? The best place to start is with your health care provider or primary care physician. They will explore your symptoms and make the referral. Ask for several referrals. Depending on your concern, you may want a therapist of a specific gender or age. A mental health professional can help you think through difficult problems that you manage on a daily basis. You will probably want to choose a therapist who has experience with diabetes.

There are many types of therapists. Therapists include psychiatrists, clinical psychologists, and clinical social workers. A psychiatrist can prescribe medications. If you have symptoms of depression, your primary care physician or therapist may prescribe an antidepressant for relief of the symptoms along with counseling.

Another consideration to think about is your health insurance. Many insurance plans provide coverage for mental health services. You can check your insurance policy for a list of benefits and providers. Compare the providers for your plan with the list given to you by your health care provider before you call to make your appointment. You may even wish to bring your insurance plan list of providers to your next routine visit to ask for a recommendation proactively.

An important tool for successful and healthy coping is your diabetes self-management plan, which will incorporate many of the self-care behaviors you have been asked to do and will be asked to do over time. It is an excellent way to make sure you are receiving the best care and allows for changes along the way. The plan should include your goals, give direction for your actions, and will make decisions easier as problems arise. Your plan will include what you know about yourself, what you know about diabetes, and jointly determine behavioral goals for you.

You and your team will work together to develop your individualized diabetes self-management plan. Everyone needs a plan, whether you are newly diagnosed or have had diabetes for a long time. Your plan will help direct your visits with your health care team. You are the most important person on that team. Remember that YOU are the expert on YOU. Taking charge of the development of your plan will help you to maintain positive health behaviors.

Some recommendations from your diabetes care team will be easier than others to incorporate into your lifestyle. Some of the self-care tasks are critical to your current and future health. You may need help prioritizing what is most important. Once you and the team are in agreement, you can work on goal setting. When developing the plan with your team, ask yourself the following questions:

- What aspect of self-care do you want to focus on?

- Are the goals written and are they clear?

- How are you going to reach the target goal?

You and your team with translate the goal into clear actionable steps. Each step will move you toward your chosen goal. A successful plan will incorporate elements of diabetes self-management education, including assessment, planning, implementation, and evaluation.

Periodically, as you work on targeted goals, you will need to determine or assess if this plan is working for you. Assessment is the cornerstone of the self-management process. If you are keeping a journal of your diabetes self-care, it becomes a great tool for assessment and problem solving. Recording successes or issues often clarifies problems in a fashion that does not happen when you are just discussing an issue. Reassessment allows for the development of realistic and achievable goals for your care.

With this information, a new plan of action may be developed. The plan is an agreement determined with your team on what you need to change. If you have had diabetes for many years you may be satisfied with your goals. In that case, the goal will remain the same. The next step is implementation. For the newly diagnosed, it may mean self-management education since there are a number of activities for which you will need to develop skills. For example, meet with the dietitian to learn how to count carbohydrates. For those who have had diabetes for a while, it may mean reviewing sick day guidelines. The final step is evaluation. Evaluation allows the team to learn if the plan and intervention were appropriate and if they achieved the desired outcome.

Take charge of your diabetes management. Actively participate in developing a care plan, learn new skills, communicate with the team your successes with self-care, and seek assistance as necessary. Your team is there to make you successful in meeting your goals for a healthy lifetime.

POSITIVE STEPS TO
HEALTHY COPING

Whether you are newly diagnosed or have had diabetes for many years, you may feel that family or friends who do not have diabetes cannot understand how you are feeling. If you have recently been diagnosed, you may feel totally overwhelmed with everything you are being instructed to do. If you have had diabetes for several years, you may be concerned because you have started to develop some complications. For many with diabetes, meeting, talking, and connecting with others can be a liberating experience. Knowing that others deal with similar challenges will validate your thoughts. If you need to connect with others with diabetes, a support group may be the answer.

There are a number of support groups available in most communities. There are support groups for different age groups or types of treatments (type 2, type 1, or insulin pump therapy). Other groups may address the needs of different population groups or those with special needs. Your diabetes educator or care team member can tell you about support groups in your area. Support groups maintain personal contact, can provide information, and act as a clearing house of experiences. Support groups will have some ground rules. They are open to free expression without criticism or interruptions. Support groups are a safe environment to express how you are feeling. To find local support groups, check your local papers for announcements of meetings, or call your local hospital.

You can also call your local American Diabetes Association (ADA) affiliate to find support groups in your area. If you live in an area without regular support groups or you are home bound, you can still connect with others via the ADA website, www.diabetes.org.

CHAPTER 8 — Successful Risk Reduction

Type 2 diabetes was once thought to be a milder form of insulin-dependent diabetes. It was referred to as "a little sugar, a touch of diabetes, or borderline diabetes". This minimized the importance of type 2 as a health concern. As recently as a decade ago, the treatment of type 2 was limited to diet, exercise, insulin, or one class of oral medications.

Today, after a decade of research, we have a much better understanding of type 2 diabetes. People with type 2 are affected with the same chronic issues as type 1. Most morbidity associated with type 2 is the result of the long-term consequences of hyperglycemia. Research has demonstrated that improved blood glucose control in type 2 diabetes reduces the rate of microvascular and macrovascular complications. Initiation of medication should begin earlier, not after failure of life-style interventions of meal planning and physical activity.

Blood glucose management of type 2 should include treating both underlying problems of insulin resistance and inadequate insulin production. The addition of insulin therapy should begin earlier in the course of treatment if target glucose levels are not met. It is estimated that 50% of those with type 2 will eventually require insulin therapy. Insulin therapy for type 2 usually begins with the introduction of basal insulin or background insulin then followed by meal coverage if needed.

The first goal of therapy is to eliminate the symptoms of hyperglycemia and optimize blood glucose control. Diabetes is diagnosed based on blood glucose level, but glucose is not the only concern in diabetes. High blood pressure and high blood cholesterol and triglycerides will lead to complications. The goals of therapy are to prevent or detect and then treat the microvascular and macrovascular complications to ensure health and well-being.

Most long-term complications develop over 10 or more years, which may seem like a long time if you were recently diagnosed. However, because of the natural history of diabetes, hyperglycemia has probably been present for 7–10 years prior to the diagnosis. Many newly diagnosed individuals present with a complication of diabetes. Often, it is the complication, not high blood glucose, that is a clue leading to the diagnosis of diabetes.

Uncontrolled blood glucose levels can take their toll over time, leading to cardiovascular complications, blindness, kidney failure, and nerve damage. The key to living well with diabetes is to reduce your risk of developing the complications associated with diabetes. Many of these complications can be prevented or delayed by focusing on reducing the risk factors. Diabetes care is a process that evolves

AMERICAN DIABETES ASSOCIATION STANDARDS OF CARE

The Standards of Care focus on all aspects of your diabetes treatment and are broken down by how often your vital body functions should be checked by your health care team.

At every visit, your health care provider:

- **Should check your blood pressure.** Your blood pressure number shows the force of blood flow through your vessels. The higher the number the harder your heart is working.

- **Should check your weight.** Weight loss may be a part of your diabetes plan. Losing as little as 10 to 15 pounds can make it easier to reach your target goals.

- **Should discuss the risks of smoking if you are a smoker.** Smoking increases the risks for heart disease, along with eye, kidney, and nerve damage.

- **Should review your blood glucose numbers.** Your blood glucose number patterns are discussed for possible changes in therapy or medications.

- **Should make time to answer your questions.** Write out questions in preparation for your appointment.

At least twice a year, your health care provider:

- **Should check your A1C.** This is a blood test that reflects your average blood over the last 2–3 months. It is the big picture of how you are managing your blood glucose. You and your team should make treatment changes based on comparing your level to your target range. If you are not meeting your target, an A1C every three to four months may be necessary.

At least once a year, your health care provider:

- **Should check your cholesterol and lipid levels.** These levels are used to determine your risk of heart attack or stroke.

- **Should measure your microalbumin.** Checking for small amounts of protein in your urine reveals how well your kidneys are functioning. This is used as an indicator of kidney damage.

- **Should examine your feet.** Your feet may need to be checked more frequently if you are having foot problems. Taking your shoes and socks off when you go into the exam room will ensure that you are checked for nerve damage or other common foot problems.

- **Should examine your eyes.** Obtain a referral to an eye doctor for a dilated eye exam. A dilated eye exam requires eye drops (so that the back of your eye can be seen).

- **Should provide you with a flu vaccine.** This is to prevent you from becoming ill.

- **Should ask about the pneumonia vaccine.** This vaccine is given once before 65 years of age and again after 65 (unless you had the vaccine within the last five years).

over time. Learning about your diabetes care and the possible complications are part of that process. As you take charge of your diabetes, you will feel empowered, knowing that you are focusing on things that can make a difference. Your reward will be a lifetime of good health.

Understanding the impact of diabetes on the body has lead the American Diabetes Association to develop guidelines for care. These guidelines are called the Standards of Medical Care in Diabetes. The Standards of Care are evidence-based guidelines that provide health care professionals with methods to manage diabetes and prevent complications. Your health care professional uses the Standards of Care as a guideline for diabetes screening, detection, and management. We will be focusing on the standards for management of diabetes including the goals of treatment. Review the Standards of Care to ensure that you are obtaining the best care possible.

People with diabetes should see their health care provider every three to six months for prevention and management. This varies depending on the type of diabetes, duration of your diabetes, your general health, how well you are meeting your therapeutic goals, and other medical conditions. Your health care providers will determine the frequency of your visits.

The Standards of Care are the cornerstones to decreasing your risk of the development of long-term complications of diabetes. The Standards focus on those areas that are evidenced to make a difference in control and prevention.

For successful risk reduction to prevent complications, you must clearly understand your target goals. The target goals are individualized numbers determined by your health care providers that keep you in optimal health. If you are unsure of your target goals, be sure to ask at your next health care appointment.

The ADA Standards of Care make recommendations of target goals for adults with diabetes. These targets are based on clinical research that determines the numbers that decrease your risk of complications, making a lifetime of good health possible. The recommendations for goals are:

- A1C of less than 7%

- A fasting glucose of 70–130 mg/dL

- A post-meal glucose of less than 180 mg/dL

- Blood pressure less than 130/80

- LDL cholesterol less than 100 mg/dL

- HDL cholesterol greater than 40 mg/dL in men and 50 mg/dL in women

- Triglyceride levels less than 150 mg/dL

The results of these tests provide an assessment and monitoring of your risks for developing complications over time. If you have your lab values recorded, you can compare them to the ADA target goals. Don't worry if you have numbers outside these recommendations; use this information to discuss treatment options with your diabetes care team. Together you will work to develop goals and actions aimed at decreasing your risks.

After recognizing that your numbers are not in line with your targeted goals or ADA recommendations, you may ask, "How can I improve those numbers to reduce my risks?" Use this question to open communications with your health care team. Your team will help you take action to bring levels into target ranges. These actions will likely include lifestyle modifications, such as healthy eating, regular physical activity, maintaining a healthy weight, and quitting smoking. If lifestyle changes don't lead to improvements, you may require medication to get your glucose, blood pressure, and cholesterol to target levels.

Healthy eating is vital for everyone. Good nutrition is the cornerstone of care for people with diabetes. Good nutrition provides the building blocks for abundant health. Think of your meals as part of your treatment plan. If you haven't met with a dietitian to design an individualized meal plan, ask you diabetes care team for a referral. Work with a registered dietitian who specializes in diabetes.

In general, the dietitian will make recommendations that include increasing fiber in your meal plan, which will help to lower blood cholesterol levels. Foods high in fiber include fruit, vegetables, whole-grain breads and cereals, oatmeal, oat bran, beans, and peas. Controlling your fat intake can also improve your cholesterol levels. Fat should account for no more than 30% of your total energy intake. Most of your fat intake should be monounsaturated or polyunsaturated. Your dietitian will help you limit the amount of saturated fat, trans fat, and cholesterol you are eating, thus lowering your blood cholesterol. If you need to improve your blood pressure, reducing your sodium intake may be recommended. Healthier meal plans should also improve your blood glucose control.

Another lifestyle modification is increasing your physical activity. Regular physical activity or exercise can improve blood glucose control, help control body weight, improve your sense of well-being,

BEST PRACTICES TO DECREASE YOUR RISKS

To improve your A1C, you should:

- Exercise regularly 4–5 times a week, for example 30 minutes each day.

- Pay attention to portions of the foods you eat.

- Increase your dose of diabetes medication or add another medication.

To improve your blood pressure, you should:

- Stop smoking.

- Reduce stress.

- Exercise, adding aerobic exercise 4–5 days a week for 30 minutes.

- Restrict high-sodium foods to lower your overall salt intake.

- Learn to check and record your blood pressure at home.

- Add a blood pressure medication.

To improve lipids, you should:

- Look at the amount and types of fat you are eating.

- Eat more of the good fats (olive oil and canola oil, fish and nuts).

- Exercise, adding aerobics 4–5 days a week for 30 minutes.

- Add a lipid-lowering medication.

To improve microalbumin, you should:

- Lower blood pressure.

- Lower A1C.

- Add blood pressure medications that are protective of kidneys.

To improve eye health, you should:

- Have regular annual eye exams.

- Improve A1C.

- Lower blood pressure.

---

and reduce risks for heart disease. General recommendations include 150 minutes of moderate activity spread over three days a week. In addition, people with type 2 are encouraged to do resistance exercise, targeting all major muscle groups at least twice a week. Consult with your health care provider to determine if you have any medical reasons not to begin an exercise program.

The good news is, the same treatment activity may improve several of your targets at the same time because diabetes complications are interconnected. It just takes a few small steps. Adding recommended exercise and making healthier food choices will improve your A1C, blood pressure, eye health, and lipid levels. Use this simple problem-solving chart (Decreasing Your Risks) to help improve your control, lower your numbers to target values, and decrease your risks.

If lifestyle modifications do not lower your cholesterol, triglycerides, and blood pressure, ask your health care team about medications to help decrease your risks. The enemy is the development of long-term complications, so do what you can to keep those complications at a minimum. If you have developed complications, actively treat with lifestyle modification, medications, and regular appointments with your health care team.

WEEK 3

Cardiovascular disease is the leading cause of death in people with diabetes. It is two to four times greater in people with diabetes than the general population. Cardiovascular disease includes both heart and blood vessel disease. You are at a higher risk for heart disease if you have uncontrolled blood glucose, because high blood glucose levels contribute to the development of fatty deposits in your blood vessels. This is called atherosclerosis, or hardening of the arteries. This limits the flow of blood to the heart, brain, and limbs. Other heart and vessel diseases include:

- Coronary artery disease (clogged arteries to the heart), which can cause heart attack or chest pain due to restricted blood flow.

- Congestive heart failure (heart pumps less blood than the body needs).

- Stroke, which causes death of brain cells due to clogged blood vessels or bleeding.

- Peripheral vascular disease (in which leg arteries become blocked, not allowing enough blood to pass), which causes pain.

In addition to hyperglycemia, other cardiovascular risk factors include: family history, carrying extra weight around your waist (apple shape), high blood pressure, high cholesterol, high LDL cholesterol, high triglycerides, and low HDL cholesterol.

Prevention behaviors are the things you can do now to avoid cardiovascular disease. To reduce your risk factors, change your lifestyle behaviors. Begin by increasing your physical activity. Keep your A1C at the target of <7%, check your blood glucose regularly with self-blood glucose monitoring, and maintain a healthy body weight. Another factor in heart disease is high cholesterol. High LDL cholesterol and triglycerides and low HDL cholesterol are common in diabetes. Controlling your cholesterol can reduce your risk of a heart attack or stroke by 20–50%. Be sure to follow a healthy meal plan that is high in fiber and low in fat. Have your blood pressure checked at every health care visit. The goal is 130/80 mmHg or less. Controlling your blood pressure lowers your risk of heart disease or stroke by 33–50%. Blood pressure within target levels will reduce your chances of developing eye, kidney, or nerve diseases by 33%. It's easy to see how a few modifiable lifestyle changes can successfully reduce your risk of complications.

Sometimes even with your best efforts, you may require medication to lower levels within target range. Even when LDL levels are on target, the ADA recommends statin therapy for anyone who has diabetes and is 40 years or older. Statins are a group of medications that lower the risk of heart attack and stroke. It may require several medications with the addition of ACE inhibitors or angiotensin receptor blockers (ARBs). Sometimes it will take a combination of medication to control your blood pressure and lipids.

Studies have shown that aspirin can prevent heart disease from developing in those at high risk. Ask your health care provider if you should take low dose aspirin daily. There are a number of things to consider before you begin taking aspirin. Although aspirin is over the counter, it does not mean it comes without risks. A low dose of 81–325 mg is recommended because it has fewer side effects. Aspirin therapy is recommended for most adults over 30 years of age with diabetes to improve blood flow. Talk with your health care provider about any concerns you may have when taking medications.

Renal disease is a disease of the kidneys. The kidneys are two bean shaped organs in the middle of your back. They contain a million tiny filtering units called nephrons that remove the waste from the blood. The useful components like protein and red blood cells remain in the blood, while the rest becomes waste and is excreted as urine. Diabetes can damage kidneys, making them less efficient. Over time, high levels of blood glucose cause the kidneys to filter too much blood. The kidneys work overtime to remove wastes from building up in the blood, and eventually stop working properly. Useful proteins are lost to the urine. A simple lab test can detect early signs of kidney disease. Your health care provider will want to measure the amount of protein albumin in your urine annually. Subtle increases in mircoalbuminuria indicate early kidney damage. Once protein is detected, there are many treatment options to prevent or slow the progression of kidney damage.

Renal disease is not inevitable, because kidney disease progresses slowly. One of the earliest symptoms of renal disease is fluid build up (edema), often in the abdomen and chest and around the heart. The build up of fluid may cause fatigue, shortness of breath, or frequent urination. Many notice their shoes and clothes feel tight because of edema. By the time symptoms are present, the kidneys have already suffered injury and damage.

Other symptoms that develop as the disease advances include:

- Loss of appetite

- Feeling cold

- Poor concentration

- Nausea

- Itching

As the disease advances vomiting, bruising, weight loss, daytime sleepiness, insomnia, muscle cramps, and restless leg may occur.

To keep your kidneys healthy, maintain blood glucose levels as close to normal as possible. Following your meal plan, getting regular exercise, taking your medications, and monitoring your glucose with SBGM will improve glucose control. See your diabetes care team on a regular basis to monitor your A1C, blood pressure, and test your urine for protein.

If you have kidney problems, controlling blood glucose and blood pressure can slow and even reverse the damage. Other lifestyle modifications include having a balanced meal plan low in cholesterol and limiting your intake of sodium. When you have renal problems, consulting with a dietitian is necessary because you may be asked to make adjustments in sodium and protein, making your meal plans a little more complex. Avoid smoking and alcohol use.

When you have kidney problems you may be instructed to limit your use of supplements and over-the-counter drugs. Always make sure your health care providers are aware of your medications by taking your medication list to all appointments. Some common medications such as ibuprofen (Advil, Motrin, and generic brands) and naproxen (Aleve) can cause damage to the kidneys. Be aware that injected dyes used in some x-ray procedures can cause kidney failure a few days later, so always make sure x-ray technicians know you have kidney disease. They will give you fluids and drugs to reduce your risks.

Your health care providers will discuss the addition of medications to lower blood pressure, protect, and slow the progression of kidney disease. The addition of an angiotensin-converting enzyme inhibitor (ACE) or angiotensin receptor blocker (ARB) may be prescribed. Both pills lower blood pressure and slow kidney disease.

If kidney problems progress and the kidneys lose filtering ability, you will need to have another way to clean waste from the blood. Kidney dialysis or a kidney transplant are treatment options that may be necessary if the disease has progressed. One dialysis option is hemodialysis, a procedure with an artificial kidney machine that you are attached to three times a week for 3–6 hours. This machine will filter waste from your blood and return it clean to your body. Another option is peritoneal dialysis, where a tube is inserted and fills your abdomen with a fluid called dialysate over 4–6 hours. A similar procedure can also be done while you sleep, instead of dealing with bags during the daytime.

If dialysis in not an option, you will probably need a kidney transplant. This treatment is only used for advanced kidney disease. A donor kidney is obtained and transplanted in your body. Even with immune-suppressive drugs, the body can reject the new kidney. If a kidney is rejected, it is necessary to go back to dialysis or obtain a new kidney. Awareness of a complication, receiving regular diabetes care, and self managment are the keys to delaying or preventing renal disease.

A number of eye diseases are common in those who have had long-term diabetes. Research has shown diabetes-related eye complications are preventable. Today, most people with diabetes have minor disorders. These eye complications include glaucoma, cataracts, and disorders of the retina.

Glaucoma occurs when increased pressure builds up in the eye. The pressure damages the blood vessels, decreasing blood to the optic nerve. If unchecked, the high pressure can cause loss of vision over time due to retina and nerve damage. People with diabetes are 40% more likely to develop glaucoma. Risk increases with age and duration of diabetes. There are several treatments for glaucoma, including drugs to lower eye pressure.

Cataracts are opaque areas on the lens of the eye that can impair vision if they become large enough. Cataracts are more common in people with diabetes and at younger ages. If cataracts impair vision, they may be surgically removed to restore vision. Sometimes a new transplanted lens is implanted. When the cataracts are mild, wearing sunglasses with glare-controlled lenses may help.

Diabetic retinopathy changes of the retina are caused by exposure to high blood glucose over a period of time. There are two types of retinopathy: nonproliferative and proliferative.

Nonproliferative is the most common type of retinopathy. The capillaries in the back of the eye balloon out and form pouches. Nonproliferative retinopathy usually does not require treatment. Although retinopathy does not usually cause vision loss at this stage, the changes in capillary walls may cause fluid to leak into the part of the eye where focusing occurs, causing the macula to swell. Treatment consisting of eye drops is effective at stopping and sometimes reversing vision loss. There are usually no symptoms of nonproliferative retinopathy in most people.

For some people, retinopathy progresses to proliferative retinopathy. This is more serious, and if left untreated, it may lead to blindness. With proliferative retinopathy, the blood vessels become damaged, causing them to close off. In response to the decrease in blood supply, new vessels start to grow in the retina. The new vessels are weak and can leak blood into the eye, blocking vision. New blood vessels can cause scar tissue to grow, distorting or detaching the retina. Unfortunately, the retina can be badly damaged before you notice any changes in vision. Many people have no symptoms with proliferative retinopathy until it is too late, so be sure to have regular eye exams even if you have not noticed any problems. Early detection is important if you are experiencing eye changes. Many advances have been made in laser surgery, which has been shown to lower your risk of severe vision loss or blindness.

There are a number of interventions to avoid vision loss. Have a dilated eye exam performed by an ophthalmologist or optometrist to preserve vision. With type 2 diabetes, you should have the exam at diagnosis because of the natural progression of diabetes and exposure to elevated blood glucose for years prior to diagnosis. After the initial exam, have a dilated eye exam annually. If you have eye disease, you may need an exam more frequently if recommended. Make lifestyle interventions to improve blood glucose control and blood pressure control to reach your target range. An annual eye exam for early detection, improving blood glucose, and blood pressure control will decrease your risks for developing eye disease by an estimated 50–60%.

Neuropathy is any disease of the nerves. Nerves are responsible for messages to and from the brain telling muscles how and when to move. Nerves also communicate sensations of temperature, touch, or pain. Nerves control genitourinary, gastrointestinal, cardiovascular, and other body functions. Nerve damage from diabetes is called diabetic neuropathy, and it is estimated that 60–70% of people with diabetes have a mild to severe form of nerve damage. Diabetic neuropathy is a very common complication of diabetes. The development of diabetic neuropathy is related to the duration of diabetes, and can cause long-term complications.

The two common types of neuropathy are peripheral neuropathy and autonomic neuropathy. Peripheral neuropathy, or sensorimotor neuropathy, causes tingling, numbness, weakness, or pain in your feet and hands. Autonomic neuropathy affects the nerves that control your bladder, intestines, genitals, and cardiovascular system. Autonomic neuropathies have symptoms of urinary frequency, bladder emptying and urinary tract infections, impotence, decreased vaginal lubrication and frequency of orgasm, early feeling of fullness when eating, after-meal low blood glucose, fainting, loss of warning signs of a heart attack, and increased or decreased sweating, to name a few.

Many of the symptoms of neuropathy can be caused by something else, making diagnosis often a challenge. Assessment during a complete physical exam includes: the evaluation of sensation, temperature, position, muscle strength and deep tendon reflexes confirm the diagnosis.

You can prevent or delay nerve damage. If you are diagnosed with diabetic neuropathy, there are a number of treatments to decrease the symptoms of neuropathy. One treatment method will not be effective in everyone. Treatment for neuropathy is individualized, so you may need to try more than one for relief. Treatment options for diabetic neuropathy are focused on blood glucose control, pain management, relief from depression often found with chronic pain, and protecting

COULD YOU HAVE DIABETIC NEUROPATHY AND NOT KNOW IT?

If you have diabetes and are experiencing any of the following symptoms, talk to your doctor right away. All of these could be early signs of neuropathy.

- My feet tingle.
- I feel "pins and needles" in my feet.
- I have burning, stabbing, or shooting pains in my feet.
- My feet are very sensitive to touch. For example, it hurts to have bed covers touch my feet.
- My feet hurt at night.
- My feet and hands get very cold or very hot.
- My feet are numb and feel dead.
- I don't feel pain in my feet, even when I have blisters or injuries.
- I can't feel my feet when I'm walking.
- The muscles in my feet and legs are weak.
- I'm unsteady when I stand or walk.
- I have trouble feeling heat or cold in my feet or hands.
- I have open sores (ulcers) on my feet and legs. These sores heal very slowly.
- It seems like the muscles and bones in my feet have changed shape.

American Diabetes Association Website: www.diabetes.org/type-2-diabetes/diabetic-neuropathy.jsp. Accessed December 2, 2007.

feet from injury. Neuropathy causes impaired sensation, leading to a loss of feeling in your feet, legs, hands, or arms. This insensitivity to pain will often mean a cut or wound will go unnoticed, perhaps leading to infection, ulceration, and amputation. Keep your blood glucose levels in the target range. Healthy meal plans, physical activity, and taking your medications will help you reach an A1C < 7%. If you are not achieving target range, you are placing yourself at risk for developing neuropathies. Use the checklist at left; making a list of your signs and symptoms. If you are having symptoms, report these to your health care provider as soon as possible. Early interventions can stop further problems from developing.

Severe forms of diabetic neuropathy are a contributing factor in the development of lower-extremity amputations. We know hyperglycemia and neuropathic pain are predictive of ulcers and amputations. Amputation rates for people with diabetes are 10 times higher than for the general population. Although the risk is greater for amputations, studies have shown daily simple self-foot exams can reduce amputation rates by 45–85%.

An annual comprehensive foot examination should be done at your health care visit. A comprehensive exam will include the health care provider using a monofilament (small nylon strand), a tuning fork, palpation (touching), checking pulses, and a visual examination. Your feet should be checked at each visit. Taking your shoes and socks off in the exam room will help remind your health care provider to check your feet. Be sure to point out any area of concern, such as sensitivity, pain, or a cut or sore that has not healed.

To prevent foot complications, take care of your feet every day. Foot care is a self-care skill you will want to develop because it's the easiest way to detect risk factors earlier, preventing serious complications.

- Look for breaks or cuts in the skin.

- Look for sores, cuts, bumps, dry skin, corns, calluses, blisters, reddened areas, swelling, ingrown toenails, and toenail infections.

- Observe for any swelling.

- Look for reddened areas.

- Touch your foot to feel for hot areas.

- Look between the toes.

- Place a mirror under your foot to clearly see the underside. If you are having trouble seeing, or difficulty bending, ask an educator to show you other ways you can examine your feet. You can have a family member help check.

If you find anything unusual or changes to your feet, report these to your health care team.

SUCCESSFUL RISK
REDUCTION

DAILY FOOT CARE TIPS

1. Keep feet clean. Wash them daily with warm water and a mild bar soap.

2. Don't soak unless a health care provider instructs you to.

3. Dry between toes.

4. Use lotion on top and bottom of feet, not between toes. Use a moisturizing lotion that is not perfumed or with alcohol so it is drying.

5. Wear the right shoes and socks.

6. Wear breathable materials such as leather or canvas.

7. Shoes should not be too tight, leaving pressure marks.

8. Prevent cracking of feet. This is a possible entry for bacteria.

9. Wear socks or pantyhose, not knee highs that could cause circulation problems.

10. Always wear your shoes, even indoors.

11. Check inside your shoes and socks before putting them on. Small objects, such as tacks, stones, or other objects, will break the skin if you walk around all day.

12. Avoid wearing sandals if you have neuropathy.

13. File your toenails straight across. Don't use scissors, knives, or razors, because you can cut yourself.

When you have diabetes, there are a number of skills necessary for day-to-day management. This section will cover several key areas that cross all methods of diabetes treatment and complication prevention.

Learn all you can

Diabetes Self-Management Education and Training (DSME) is an integral part of your care. Medical Nutrition Therapy (MNT) is essential to diabetes prevention, management, and self-management education. Everyone living with diabetes needs to learn all they can to effectively self-manage their diabetes. Diabetes education is essential when you are first diagnosed, and is also recommended at least annually. Meeting with your diabetes educator helps you handle changes in health status and treatment. Your diabetes will change over time. Make your appointment for a DSME and MNT consult if you have not seen an educator or dietitian in over a year. Your educators will ensure that your care is meeting the ADA Standards of Care and will review your diabetes management plan with you.

Self-monitoring blood glucose

Self-monitoring of blood glucose (SMBG) is a component of effective therapy. Results of SMBG allow people with diabetes to evaluate their response to medications, meal planning, and physical activities. The accuracy of SMBG depends on the user and instrument; therefore, it is important to be evaluated for your technique and the working order of your monitor at regular intervals. Many people with diabetes are taught to use the data to make adjustments in their meal plans, exercise, or medication. Your health care providers will evaluate your use of the data at your health care visits and will review with you your blood glucose monitoring logs for patterns in high and low readings. Those patterns are a tool to guide options for treatment decisions. Be sure to take your meter and log or record to every visit.

Maintaining personal care records

As previously discussed, developing and maintaining a record of your personal health is a valuable tool. It allows you to play an active role on your diabetes care team and in the important decisions regarding your health.

Your diabetes management plan is a part of your care records, providing you with the target ranges for each laboratory test and guidelines for therapy. Be sure to ask for your numbers at your visit with your health care provider. Keeping a record will allow you to see your improvements over time and identify areas that need continued focus.

If you are not meeting therapeutic goals, ask what you should do to meet those goals.

Sometimes, it is difficult to ask questions, or your memory slips when you are in the office. To be prepared, write questions down before your appointment. Carry a notebook and a pen so you can copy down instructions from your appointments. It can help to bring a family member to the visits, so you can be sure you heard and understood everything that is suggested. You will get the most out of your visit if you are prepared. After your visit, follow through with the suggestions your health care providers have recommended.

Monitoring blood pressure

Even mild elevations in blood pressure increase the risk of complications such as eye disease, kidney disease, and heart disease; however, research indicates that achieving your target of 130/80 mg/dL or less will give you the same protective benefit as people without diabetes. One way to improve your blood pressure is to learn more about how blood pressure affects your overall health. Ask for your blood pressure the next time it is taken in the office and write it on your tracker. If it is elevated, you may be asked to check your blood pressure at home on a regular basis and keep a record. Devices for home use are readily available and easy to use. Monitoring at home will allow you to follow your improvement and watch closely the effect of various treatment strategies, such as starting a walking program or decreasing sodium in your diet. If you are not reaching your targets, ask about medications to treat high blood pressure. Some blood pressure medications not only lower blood pressure, but help protect kidneys as well.

Prepregnancy counseling

Women with diabetes considering pregnancy need to be seen by a multidisciplinary team for evaluation. The team will advise that your A1C should be as close to normal as possible before conception. Because of this recommendation, all women with diabetes of childbearing age should be informed regarding the need for good glucose control. Contraception is suggested until normal sustained blood glucose is achieved. Those meeting with a multidisciplinary team will be evaluated and treated for long-term complications of diabetes. The team will review all medications currently taken as part of preconception care. A preconception program will train patients in diabetes self-management with diet, intensified insulin therapy as needed, and SMBG in preparation for pregnancy.

Erectile dysfunction

Sexual dysfunction is a frequent occurrence in men with diabetes. In fact, men with diabetes are twice as likely to develop erectile dysfunction (ED). ED is caused by damage to the nerves over many years, and presents with a lack of a firm and sustained erection for intercourse. In general, libido and ejaculatory function are not affected.

There may be several reasons for the development of ED. Diabetes can damage the nerves in the penis, preventing an erection, even if you are interested in sexual activity. Diabetes can also damage the blood vessels in the penis, not allowing blood to reach the area during sexual arousal, shortening the duration of the erection. Other factors can be side effects of some medications, such as high blood pressure medications, beta-blockers, or antidepressants. Alcohol, smoking, stress, and illness can also cause ED, along with conditions like prostate problems or complications from bladder surgery. Talk with your health provider if you are experiencing difficulties.

There are a variety of treatments for ED including pills (Cialis, Levitra, and Viagra), suppositories that are inserted into the tip of the penis, injections that are taken before sexual activity, and implants. Other diabetes lifestyle changes you are incorporating may also help. Couple counseling, relaxation techniques, and stress reduction techniques may decrease your anxiety about your symptoms.

CONCLUSION

Look how far you have come with your efforts to improve your lifestyle to enhance your diabetes control. It is important to pat yourself on the back for whatever changes in behavior you have made. Always, always, give yourself the credit you deserve.

Reward yourself! Think about what it would take to feel like you are receiving a reward for all of your accomplishments. Try and establish a reward system that does not keep you from focusing on your goal. For example, going to an all-you-can-eat buffet may not be the right thing to keep you on track; however, a membership to a gym or getting a massage might be just what the doctor ordered.

PARTING WORDS TO REMEMBER ABOUT SELF-CARE BEHAVIOR

- It does not promise beauty, but it will improve your health.
- It is not a quick process, but slow and methodical.
- It is not easy, but often difficult and sometimes painful.
- It does not tell you what to do, but helps you decide what is worth doing.
- It does not take responsibility for your choices, but offers information and support so you can make informed choices.
- It is not pre-packaged, but a custom-designed program for you by you.
- It does not apply external forces, but seeks to help you discover the forces within yourself.
- It does not judge your circumstances, but helps you live with them.
- It does not solve your problems, but offers tools to solve them.
- It does not simplify, but acknowledges the complexity.
- It is not an easy sell, but a path to real and lasting change.

Adapted from: Adolfsson, B, Arnold, MS. Behavioral Approaches to Treating Obesity: Some Words to Remember About Behavior Change. *American Diabetes Association, 2006. p. 138.*

Keep in mind that your lifestyle changes require day-to-day attention. Any chronic illness like diabetes is with you for life. It may be helpful to focus on one day at a time, rather than think about the rest of your life all at once. By focusing on one day at a time and your blood glucose control for today, hopefully you will be able to maintain the best possible control, as well as reward yourself.

INDEX

A

A1C levels, 8, 30, 56, 67–68, 130–131, 145

Activity, 31–50, 134. *See also Exercise*

Aerobic exercise, 33–34

Air travel, 90

Albumin, 139. *See also Microalbumin*

Alcohol use, 29, 140

Alpha-glucosidase inhibitors, 70

Alternative exercise methods, 46

Alternative site glucose testing, 61

American College of Sports Medicine, 35, 45

American Diabetes Association (ADA)

  recommendations from, 21, 31, 45, 52, 67, 138

  resources provided by, 27, 47, 103, 127

  Standards of Medical Care from, 32, 130–133, 135, 148

Amputations, 146

Aspirin therapy, 138

Autonomic neuropathy, 144

B

BC-ADM. *See Board certified-advanced diabetes management certification*

Beans, 14, 134

Behavior change, 153

Biguanides, 71, 78

Biofeedback, 118

Blindness, 130, 143

Blood glucose levels, 2–3. *See also Hyperglycemia; Hypoglycemia; Meters*

  comparing with exercise efforts, 43

  controlling, 4, 7–8, 26, 37, 51–53, 60

  losing control of, 121, 130

  managing fluctuations in, 92–93

  monitoring, 51–68

  patterns of, 62–63

  setting targets for, 105

Blood pressure

  controlling, 3, 7, 134–135, 138

  high, 129

  monitoring, 149–150

BMI. *See Body mass index*

Board certified-advanced diabetes management (BC-ADM) certification, 5

Body mass index (BMI), 9–11

  table for, 10

Body weight, healthier, 8–11

Borg Rate of Perceived Exertion, 42

Buffet eating, 28–29

C

Calories

  burning with exercise, 49

  monitoring, 16, 20

Carbohydrates

  awareness of, 11–12

  fast-acting, 39, 98–100, 107–108

  target amounts, 17–18, 25, 29

J

Journaling, 104, 106, 118, 126

K

Ketoacidosis. *See Diabetic ketoacidosis*
Ketones, testing for, 96
Kidney failure, 130. *See also Renal disease*

L

Labels. *See Food labels*
Laser surgery, 143
LDL. *See Low density lipoprotein*
Lifestyle changes, needed, 7, 109, 120, 136–137, 154
Lipids. See Fat intake
Low density lipoprotein (LDL), 11, 137
   LDL cholesterol, 32, 137

M

Managing diabetes. *See Self-management of diabetes*
Meal planning, 7–8, 28, 134, 140
Meats, 14, 29
Medical care team, 4
Medical clearance, 37–39
Medical jewelry, 107
Medical Nutrition Therapy (MNT), 148
Medical records, 84. *See also Recording blood glucose numbers*
Medications, 69–90, 136, 138. *See also Cost factors; individual medications*
   barriers to taking, 87–88
   common, 140

missing doses of, 87
side effects and interactions, 78–79
storage and disposal of, 84
taking inventory of, 76–77
types of, 70–75
Meditation, 118
Meglitinides, 71
Memory challenges, week 4, 82–83
Mental health aspects, 4, 123–124
Meters
   accuracy of, 54–55, 95
   proper use of, 61
   setting clock correctly, 63
Microalbumin, 130, 135
Milk, 14, 25
MNT. *See Medical Nutrition Therapy*
Monitoring. *See also Recording blood glucose numbers; Self-monitoring of blood glucose*
   blood glucose levels, 51–68
   blood pressure, 149–150
   calories, 16
   frequency of, 59, 65
Motivation, 112
"My Pyramid," 12–14

N

Needles, safe disposal of, 84
Negativity, 112, 121–122
Nerve damage, 130
Nerve disease, 144–147
Neuropathy, 144–147
Nursing care (RN), 4
Nutrition
   knowing the facts, 19–21
   modifying intake of, 7, 134
Nutrition Labeling and Education Act, 19

O

Online pharmacies, 86
Oral diabetes medications,
70–71, 78
combined forms, 86

P

Pedometer, 40–41
Pens, pre-filled with insulin, 73
Persistence, 47–48
Pharmacists, 84–86
online, 86
Physical activity, 33
Physical stress, 117
Physician care, 4, 37–39, 111,
123–124
Pill boxes, 82–83
Portion size, 20, 22–24, 28
doing the "hand jive," 23
Positive change, recognizing, 30,
49–50
Pramlintide, 73
Pre-filled pens, 73
Prediabetes, 2–3
Pregnancy, 151
and gestational diabetes, 2
Prescriptions, 76–77. *See also
Medications*
Prevention
of cardiovascular disease,
137–138
of diabetes, 31–32
of problems with diabetes,
92–93
of short term complications,
104
Problems with diabetes, 91–108
solving, 106
Psychological therapy, 124

R

Rate of Perceived Exertion (RPE), 42
RDs. *See Registered dietitians*
Recording blood glucose numbers,
58, 62–63, 77, 104, 149
Registered dietitians (RDs), 4, 8,
15, 17–18, 22, 28
Relaxation techniques, 118, 152
Renal disease, 139–141
Resiliency, 112
Resistance training, 34–35, 44–45.
See also Insulin resistance
Restaurant eating, 24, 27–29
Retinopathy, 142–143
Reward system, 153
Risks
cardiovascular, 137–138
reducing, 129–152
of type 2 diabetes, 2
RN. *See Nursing care*
RPE. *See Rate of Perceived Exertion*

S

Safety precautions, 34, 84,
107–108
Self-management of diabetes, 3,
56, 81, 91
education for, 5, 92, 96,
102–103
empowerment for, 113–114,
125–126
equipment for, 54, 84
lifestyle changes needed, 7,
109, 120
Self-monitoring of blood glucose
(SMBG), 148
Sharps Disposal Containers, 84
Sick day guidelines, 99–101, 105,
126

OTHER TITLES FROM THE AMERICAN DIABETES ASSOCIATION

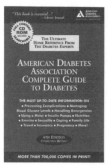

American Diabetes Association Complete Guide to Diabetes, 4th Edition
by American Diabetes Association
Have all the tips and information on diabetes that you need close at hand. The world's largest collection of diabetes self-care tips, techniques, and tricks for solving diabetes-related problems is back in its fourth edition, and it's bigger and better than ever before.
Order no. 4809-04; New low price $19.95

The Healthy Carb Diabetes Cookbook
by Chef Jennifer Bucko, MCFE, and Laura Rondinelli, RD, LDN, CDE
Worried about carbs? The 199 delicious recipes featured in *The Healthy Carb Diabetes Cookbook* prove that carbs aren't just ok—they're essential. Every recipe in this book is handcrafted by Chef Jennifer Bucko and Lara Rondinelli to be healthy and great tasting.
Order no. 4666-01; Price $18.95

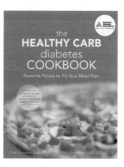

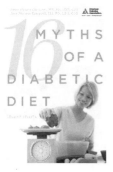

16 Myths of a Diabetic Diet
by Karen Hanson Chalmers, MS, RD, LDN, CDE, and Amy Peterson Campbell, MS, RD, LDN, CDE
16 Myths of a Diabetic Diet will tell you the truth about diabetes and how to eat when you have diabetes. Learn what the most common myths about diabetes meal plans are, where they come from, and how to overcome them. Let experts Karen Chalmers and Amy Campbell show you how to create and follow a healthy, enjoyable way of eating.
Order no. 4829-02; Price $14.95

The 4-Ingredient Diabetes Cookbook
by Nancy Hughes
Making delicious meals doesn't have to be complicated, time-consuming, or expensive. You can create satisfying dishes using just four ingredients (or even fewer)! Make the most of your time and money. You'll be amazed at how much you can prepare with just a few simple ingredients.
Order no. 4662-01; Price $16.95

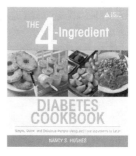

To order these and other great American Diabetes Association titles, call *1-800-232-6733* or visit *http://store.diabetes.org*.
American Diabetes Association titles are also available in bookstores nationwide.